RED CELL MANUAL

ROBERT S. HILLMAN, M.D.

and

CLEMENT A. FINCH, M.D.

Division of Hematology
Health Sciences Learning Resources Center
University of Washington Medical School
Seattle, Washington

EDITION
4

F. A. DAVIS COMPANY
PHILADELPHIA, PA.

Copyright © 1974 by F. A. Davis Company

Second printing 1974
Third printing 1975
Fourth printing 1975
Fifth printing 1976
Sixth printing 1978

ISBN 0-8036-4633-X
Library of Congress Catalog Card Number 73-88798

Printed in the United States of America

INTRODUCTION

The information presented in this manual is designed
as a guide for the general physician or for the student
developing competence in dealing with red cell disorders.
Detailed considerations of specific diseases are left to the
province of the specialist and are well described in many
standard textbooks of hematology (1,2). Part 1 of the manual
contains general concepts of normal red cell production and
destruction, oxygen transport and the effects of pathologic
mechanisms on the erythron. For amplification, the reader is
referred to the excellent books of Williams et al (1) and
Harris and Kellermeyer (3). Part 2 of the manual proposes a
logical clinical approach to red cell disorders. Part 3 is a
discussion of laboratory procedures on which this approach is
based. References are either to general reviews or to papers
in which a specific investigation documents a single point.
Acknowledgment is made of the many contributions of past
research fellows, associates and friends who have assisted in
this formulation.

CONTENTS

PART 1 - CONCEPTS

PART 2 - CLINICAL APPROACH

PART 3 - LABORATORY APPROACH

v

PART 1 CONCEPTS

I. QUALITATIVE ASPECTS OF ERYTHROPOIESIS

A. Marrow Structure

In the fetus, **erythrocyte-forming tissue** is located in the **liver, spleen and skeleton.** After birth, hematopoietic colonization of the **liver** and spleen declines. Then, as the individual grows, the medullary cavity of the skeleton enlarges, and fat replaces most of the active marrow in the peripheral skeleton. The adult distribution of **red cell marrow** is shown by Fe^{52} localization (4) to be limited to the axial skeleton and proximal ends of the long bones.

Within the marrow cavity, normal architecture consists of cords of cells radiating from bony endosteum (5). A fine structure of reticulin serves to support the hematopoietic tissue and sinusoidal vasculature. The incomplete sinusoidal walls of the normal marrow vasculature permit free exchange of plasma components such as plasma proteins, but retain the developing hematopoietic cells until their rheologic characteristics enable them to emerge through the sinusoidal wall (6). The milieu provided by normal stroma appears essential for red cell development, since transplantation of marrow

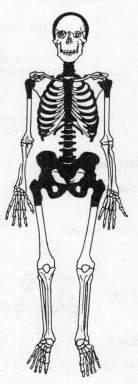

RED CELL MARROW DISTRIBUTION
IN THE ADULT

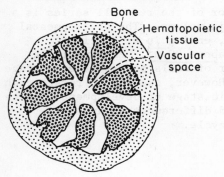

NORMAL MARROW ARCHITECTURE

Bone

Hematopoietic tissue

Vascular space

into patients with myelofibrosis is unsuccessful unless the fibrotic tissue is first removed by curettage (7). When disease involves the stroma, or with extramedullary erythropoiesis, orderly release is lost, and the circulating blood contains immature as well as mature elements (myelophthisic blood picture, p.58). Abnormalities in stromal architecture may be demonstrated using marrow biopsy specimens **stained for collagen and reticulin.**

1

B. Red Cell Generation

The red cell is one of a number of cell species which originate from stem cells (cells capable of generating a self-maintaining clone). The "uncommitted" or pluripotential stem cell probably has morphological characteristics resembling those of the mature lymphocyte (8), although it cannot be identified in the marrow film. Its presence is demonstrated by the development of tumor-like clones of hematopoietic tissue in the spleen of a marrow-transfused recipient animal whose own marrow has been ablated by radiation; each clone is the progeny of a single stem cell (9). Usually quiescent, the pluripotential cell constitutes a cell-generating reserve which can respond to a depletion of "committed" stem cells, the next stage in the developmental sequence. The "committed" or unipotential stem cell, still not morphologically recognizable, is normally part of a self-perpetuating precursor pool specific for each cell line (erythrocytic, granulocytic-monocytic, megakaryocytic). Abnormalities of proliferation may result from disorders in number or behavior of these stem cells (10), although at present this is more conceptual than of practical import.

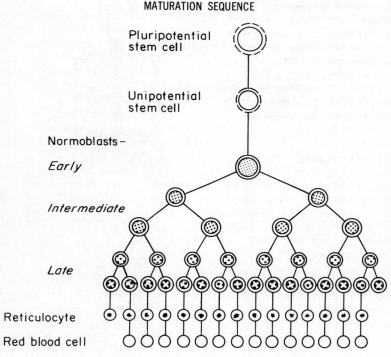

MATURATION SEQUENCE

Pluripotential stem cell

Unipotential stem cell

Normoblasts –

Early

Intermediate

Late

Reticulocyte

Red blood cell

| Erythroid Maturation Sequence |

The first recognizable ancestor of the red cell series is a large immature cell about 800 μ^3 in volume. The developmental sequence involves several mitoses, ending in an anucleate, hemoglobin-loaded erythrocyte of about 90 μ^3. Presumably, a logarithmic increase in the number of cells occurs at each stage of development up to the terminal normoblast. However, one cannot relate each of these levels of mitosis to a specific morphologic stage of development because of the continuity of the cytoplasmic maturation and differences in nuclear appearance imposed by the phase of the mitotic cycle.

To characterize the stages of red cell development and to provide a baseline for detection of abnormalities, it is convenient to divide nucleated red cells into 1) early, 2) intermediate and 3) late forms. Early forms (pro- and basophilic normoblasts) on the Wright-stained blood smear appear as large cells with pale to dark blue cytoplasm. Nuclear chromatin is slightly clumped and heavier than in the white cell series at corresponding stages of maturation; nucleoli are partially obscured by the heavy chromatin. The intermediate stage of development is characterized by a more compact nucleus and the presence of hemoglobin within the cytoplasm. Cytoplasmic color ranges from blue to gray (polychromatic normoblast) according to the amount of hemoglobin present. In the late stage of maturation, the nucleus becomes progressively smaller and just before its extrusion, is a structureless pyknotic mass. The numerical ratio of the early, intermediate and late normoblasts is approximately 1:4:4. The cytoplasm of the anucleate cell which then remains (marrow reticulocyte) shows a blue-staining net of precipitated RNA (reticulum) after treatment with a supravital dye such as new methylene blue. This cell continues to synthesize hemoglobin but at a decreased rate as it loses RNA and mitochondria and progressively shrinks in size. When it finally enters the circulation by penetrating the sinusoidal wall, the normal reticulocyte is indistinguishable from the adult red cell in size and color, but a small amount of residual RNA is still demonstrable by supravital staining. Thus, the newly circulating red cell carries a recognizable tag of its youth.

Hemoglobin is synthesized through most of the maturation process, about 65% being made before the nucleus is extruded and 35% in the reticulocyte stage (11). Normal hemoglobin production is dependent on an adequate iron supply, as well as the synthesis of protoporphyrin and globin.

Hemoglobin Synthesis

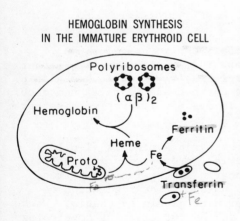

HEMOGLOBIN SYNTHESIS
IN THE IMMATURE ERYTHROID CELL

Iron is delivered by the specific transport protein, transferrin, to the membrane of the immature cell, where the iron is affixed and the transferrin released back to the plasma. Most of the iron entering the cell is committed to hemoglobin synthesis and proceeds to mitochondria where it is inserted into the protoporphyrin ring to form heme. Some excess iron accumulates as ferritin aggregates in the cytoplasm of the immature red cell where it may be demonstrated as one or more blue dots by Prussian Blue stain. The amount of non-heme iron deposited depends on the ratio between plasma iron level and the iron required by the cell for hemoglobin synthesis (12).

Porphyrin synthesis begins in the mitochondria with the formation of delta-aminolevulinic acid (ALA) and continues in the cytoplasm with the combination of two molecules of ALA to form porphobilinogen (PBG). Four molecules of PBG are converted into uroporphrinogen and coproporphrinogen. The final steps, carried

3

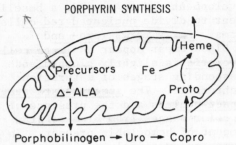

Succinate + glycine

PORPHYRIN SYNTHESIS

out in the mitochondria, involve the formation of protoporphyrin and the incorporation of iron to form heme. The most important rate-limiting step in this pathway is the conversion of succinate and glycine to delta-aminolevulinic acid, a reaction catalyzed by ALA synthetase. The activity of this enzyme is influenced by erythropoietin and by the presence of the cofactor, pyridoxal phosphate.

The polypeptide chains of globin are produced on their specific cytoplasmic ribosomes. The alpha polypeptide chain unites with one of three other chains to form a dimer and ultimately a tetramer. The normal synthesis of polypeptide chains and their respective tetramers is shown in the accompanying figure. While the γ polypeptide chain is of functional significance during fetal

FORMATION OF NORMAL HEMOGLOBINS

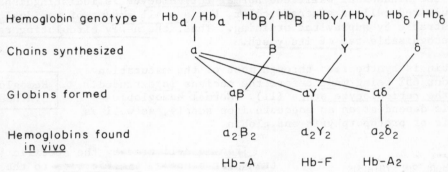

development, its persistence implies a genetic impairment in hemoglobin A production. Thus, in the thalassemias, where there is interference with either α or β formation, increased amounts of fetal hemoglobin ($\alpha_2\gamma_2$) or A_2 hemoglobin ($\alpha_2\delta_2$) or hemoglobin H (β_4) may be found. Rarely an increase in fetal hemoglobin or hemoglobin H occurs as an acquired phenomenon in myeloproliferative disorders and refractory anemias.

Globin synthesis is highly coordinated with porphyrin synthesis (1-p.101). When globin synthesis is impaired (as in thalassemia), protoporphyrin synthesis is correspondingly reduced. Similarly, when porphyrin synthesis is impaired, excess globin is not produced. However, there is no such fine regulation of iron uptake with impairment of either protoporphyrin or globin synthesis. When globin production is deficient, iron accumulates in the cytoplasm of developing red cells as ferritin aggregates. Such cells contain 2 to 10 iron-staining particles and are referred to as ferritin sideroblasts. When porphyrin synthesis is impaired, the mitochondria become encrusted with iron, and some

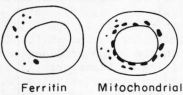

SIDEROBLASTS

Ferritin deposits   Mitochondrial loading

10 to 20 small iron-staining granules are visible around the nucleus of the developing red cell. Such a cell is called a mitochondrial or ring sideroblast. The structural difference of these iron deposits is apparent by electron microscopy; with light microscopy the distinction must be based on the number and location of granules.

C. The Adult Red Cell

The normal adult red cell is a biconcave disc, with an average diameter of 8 μ, a thickness of 2 μ, and a volume of 90 μ^3. About 33% of its volume consists of hemoglobin, which performs the function of gas (O_2 and CO_2) transport.

Hemoglobin has a molecular weight of 68,000. Due to its multichain structure the molecule is capable of considerable allosteric change as it loads and unloads O_2 (1-p.144, 13).

Hemoglobin Function

When the individual heme groups unload O_2, the beta chains are pulled apart, permitting the entrance of 2,3-diphosphoglycerate (DPG) and the establishment of salt bridges between the individual chains, resulting in a progressively lower affinity of hemoglobin for O_2. With O_2 uptake, salt bonds are broken sequentially, beta chains are pulled together expelling DPG, and the affinity of hemoglobin for O_2 is progressively increased. This "respiratory movement" between the relaxed and constricted state is responsible for the sigmoid form of the hemoglobin O_2 dissociation curve.

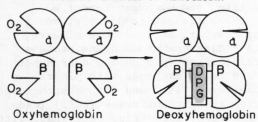

MOLECULAR CHANGES OF HEMOGLOBIN

Oxyhemoglobin   Deoxyhemoglobin

Hemoglobin affinity for O_2 is portrayed by this curve or by the expression P_{50}, which designates the partial pressure of O_2 at which hemoglobin is half-saturated under standard in vitro conditions of temperature and pH. The P_{50} of normal blood is 26.6 mm Hg. With an increase in hemoglobin affinity for O_2, the dissociation curve shifts to the left, i.e., the P_{50} falls. A decrease in affinity for O_2 is reflected in a right shift of the dissociation curve and an increase in P_{50}. Normally, in vivo O_2 exchange operates between 95% saturation (arterial blood) with a mean arterial O_2 tension of 95 mm Hg, and 70% saturation (venous blood) with a mean venous O_2 tension of 40 mm Hg.

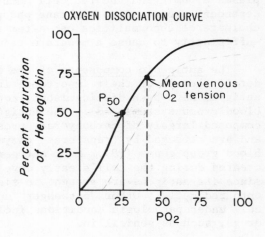

OXYGEN DISSOCIATION CURVE

Percent saturation of Hemoglobin

P_{50}

Mean venous O_2 tension

PO_2

5

↑ DPG → restrain the Hb-molecule in the deoxygenated form → ↓ Hb affinity for O_2

The normal position of the O_2 dissociation curve depends on three different ligands normally found within the red cell: H ions, CO_2 and organic phosphates (14). Of these, DPG plays the most important physiologic role (p. 9). High concentrations of these ligands restrain the hemoglobin molecule in the deoxygenated form, thereby decreasing hemoglobin affinity for O_2 and shifting the O_2 dissociation curve to the right. Alterations in the amino acid sequence of the hemoglobin molecule are also important in modifying O_2 transport (15). Fetal hemoglobin, for example, has a slightly decreased intrinsic affinity for oxygen, but due to a reduced interaction with organic phosphates has an overall increased affinity for O_2 in vivo. A variety of genetic hemoglobin abnormalities may distort the molecular structure or impose restriction on the "respiratory movement" of the hemoglobin molecule; as a result, hemoglobin affinity is either increased or decreased. Other genetic abnormalities in amino acid sequence of the hemoglobin molecule may affect O_2 transport by causing the oxidation of heme iron to methemoglobin. The clinical implications in terms of O_2 transport are discussed elsewhere (p. 22).

Erythrocyte Membrane

The red cell membrane is a bilaminar structure as seen by electron microscopy. Its chemical composition is 10% carbohydrate, 40% lipid and 50% protein. The outer hydrophilic layer contains glycolipid, glycoprotein and protein. The central hydrophobic layer contains alpha helical protein, cholesterol and phospholipids. An inner hydrophilic layer contains protein and glycoprotein. Stromal protein is made during early red cell development and lasts through its life span. While a portion of the membrane may be lost without cell destruction, new membrane cannot be produced. The membrane protein has not been characterized completely, and its role in disease is not yet fully established; however, at least one disease, hereditary spherocytosis, probably represents a disorder of membrane protein (16). Membrane lipids are affected by general changes in body lipid transport. Cholesterol comprises 25% of membrane lipid and is in exchange with plasma cholesterol. An increase in free plasma cholesterol, as found with obstructive jaundice, or a decrease in lecithin:cholesterol acetyltransferase (LCAT) leads to cholesterol accumulation on the red cell membrane, distorting cell shape with targeting and spicule formation (17). Fatty acids freely exchange between plasma albumin and the red cell membrane and are incorporated through an energy-dependent process into membrane phospholipid. Both plasma phospholipid and cholesterol abnormalities can alter the composition of the red cell membrane sufficiently to cause a moderate reduction in red cell life span.

The antigenic components of the red cell membrane have been studied in detail because of their importance in transfusion therapy. Over 100 red cell antigens have been distinguished, constituting at least 15 genetically distinct blood group systems (18). The antigenic clusters on the red cell membrane are composed largely of carbohydrate prosthetic groups on protein or lipid carriers, and are attached by transferase enzymes which are protein products of individual blood group genes (19). Most antigens are intrinsic components of the membrane, created during the cell's early development; the Lewis system is an exception, since its antigens are present in tissue fluids and only secondarily adsorbed onto red cells. Other "passenger" antigens which can be collected by the red cell under pathologic conditions include bacterial polysaccharides and certain drugs, such as penicillin.

Since the plasma normally contains antibodies against the major blood group antigens (A and B), and since other antigens can stimulate allo-antibody formation, the compatibility of transfused red cells is of critical importance in blood transfusion (20). The standard laboratory procedure is to type red cells for A, B and Rh antigens, to test serum for anti-A and anti-B (back typing), and to carry out a compatibility (cross match) test in which donor cells of the same ABO and Rh types are mixed with the patient's serum. After incubation the cell suspension is observed for agglutination and tested for antibody coating with the indirect antiglobulin (Coombs) test (p. 71).

The metabolism of the anucleate red cell is more limited than that of most body cells since there is little ability to metabolize fatty acids and amino acids and no mitochondrial apparatus for oxidative metabolism (1-p.132). Energy is generated almost exclusively through the breakdown of glucose. The overall pattern of red cell glycolysis is shown in the figure on the next page. For purposes of discussion, red cell metabolism may be subdivided into the anaerobic or Embden-Meyerhof pathway and three ancillary pathways which act in different ways to maintain the function of hemoglobin. All of these processes are essential if the erythrocyte is to transport oxygen and to maintain those physical characteristics required for its survival in circulation.

> Red Cell
> Metabolism

The Embden-Meyerhof pathway is responsible for about 90% of the red cell's glucose utilization and provides essential energy for membrane maintenance. In the breakdown of a molecule of glucose to lactate, 2 moles of ATP are consumed during the hexose portion of the pathway, but 3-4 moles are generated at the triose level. It is this net gain in ATP which provides high energy phosphate for maintenance of the disc shape and flexibility of the red cell, for maintenance of membrane lipids, and for energizing the metabolic pumps controlling sodium and potassium flux. The essential role of ATP in the red cell is demonstrated in at least two conditions: 1) early cell death (hemolytic anemia) which occurs when ATP is deficient due to inherited defects in glycolysis, and 2) the loss of viability accompanying ATP depletion of blood stored in vitro (21). The Embden-Meyerhof pathway also maintains pyridine nucleotides in a reduced state to permit their function in oxidative-reductive homeostasis within the cell.

The oxidative pathway or hexose monophosphate shunt is an ancillary energy system which couples oxidative metabolism with pyridine nucleotide (TPN or NADP) and glutathione reduction. The activity of this pathway increases with increased oxidation of glutathione. When the pathway is functionally deficient the amount of reduced glutathione becomes insufficient to neutralize oxidants, causing globin denaturation and precipitation as aggregates (Heinz bodies) within the cell. These masses attach themselves to the cell membrane and are ultimately removed by the reticuloendothelial cells within the spleen along with that portion of the red cell membrane to which they are attached. If the process inflicts sufficient membrane damage, the cell is destroyed. Such oxidative destruction of red cells usually occurs episodically as the result of an increased oxidant load in an individual with a latent decrease in pathway ...acity (p. 43), but a severe enzyme defect in the oxidative pathway may in ... cause a chronic hemolytic anemia. It is clear, therefore, that some ... y in the aerobic pathway is essential for normal red cell survival.

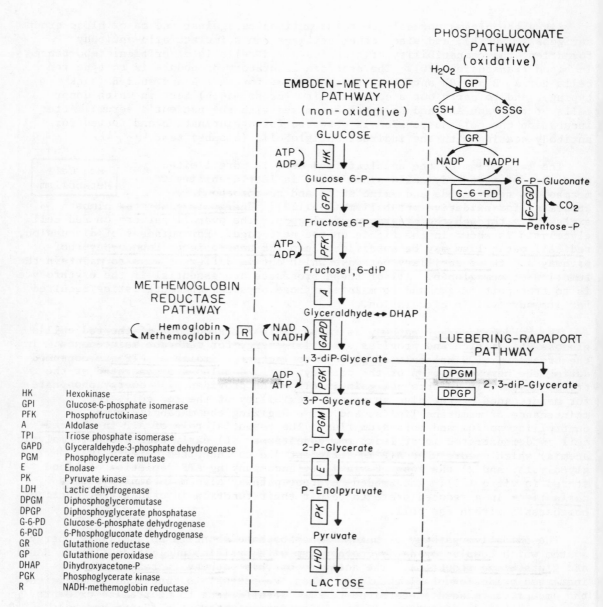

PHOSPHOGLUCONATE
PATHWAY
(oxidative)

EMBDEN–MEYERHOF
PATHWAY
(non-oxidative)

H_2O_2

GP

GSH   GSSG

GR

NADP   NADPH

GLUCOSE

ATP ⟩ HK
ADP ⟩

Glucose 6-P   6-P-Gluconate

GPI   G-6-PD   6-PGD CO_2

Fructose 6-P   Pentose-P

ATP ⟩ PFK
ADP ⟩

Fructose 1,6-diP

METHEMOGLOBIN
REDUCTASE
PATHWAY

A

Hemoglobin ⟩ R ⟩ NAD
Methemoglobin ⟩   ⟩ NADH

Glyceraldhyde ↔ DHAP

GAPD

LUEBERING–RAPAPORT
PATHWAY

1,3-diP-Glycerate

ADP ⟩ PGK
ATP ⟩

DPGM
DPGP   2,3-diP-Glycerate

3-P-Glycerate

PGM

2-P-Glycerate

E

P-Enolpyruvate

PK

Pyruvate

LHD

LACTOSE

HK	Hexokinase
GPI	Glucose-6-phosphate isomerase
PFK	Phosphofructokinase
A	Aldolase
TPI	Triose phosphate isomerase
GAPD	Glyceraldhyde-3-phosphate dehydrogenase
PGM	Phosphoglycerate mutase
E	Enolase
PK	Pyruvate kinase
LDH	Lactic dehydrogenase
DPGM	Diphosphoglyceromutase
DPGP	Diphosphoyglycerate phosphatase
G-6-PD	Glucose-6-phosphate dehydrogenase
6-PGD	6-Phosphogluconate dehydrogenase
GR	Glutathione reductase
GP	Glutathione peroxidase
DHAP	Dihydroxyacetone-P
PGK	Phosphoglycerate kinase
R	NADH-methemoglobin reductase

The methemoglobin reductase pathway is another important component of red cell metabolism. Just as there is a mechanism for protecting hemoglobin against oxidative denaturation, so there is need to prevent the oxidation of heme iron. Methemoglobin, which results from the conversion of the bivalent iron of heme to the trivalent form, can no longer combine reversibly with O_2, and O_2 transport function is lost. Maintenance of heme iron in a functional state (Fe^{++}) requires the reducing action of the pyridine nucleotide (DPN or NAD) and the enzyme methemoglobin reductase. In the absence of this system about 2% of circula hemoglobin is oxidized daily until 20-40% methemoglobin is present within cell. Nonspecific reductants in the body are sufficient to keep the remaining hemoglobin reduced. A latent deficiency of methemoglobin reductase is compatible with normal function of hemoglobin under basal conditions, but will result in high levels of methemoglobin when the individual is challenged by an oxidant drug (22).

Insight into the capacity of the normal and abnormal cell to deal with methemoglobin is gained by observing changes after hemoglobin has been converted to methemoglobin by the intravenous injection of nitrite. In normal subjects, methemoglobin will be reduced with a T 1/2 of about 120 minutes. This rate of reduction may be greatly accelerated with methylene or toluidine blue (T 1/2 of 10 minutes) since these dyes function similarly to cytochrome, coupling NADP reductase and the aerobic pathway with methemo-globin reduction. In patients with a deficiency of NAD-dependent methemoglobin reductase there is no spontaneous reversion after nitrite (23). At the same time, methylene blue or toluidine blue produces rapid reduction similar to that in the normal individual. With certain inherited abnor-malities of hemoglobin structure (M hemoglobino-pathies), these dyes are ineffective since the abnormal hemoglobins will not couple with the NADP reductase pathway (24).

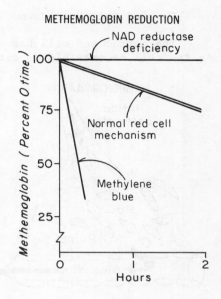

METHEMOGLOBIN REDUCTION

Confusion is often caused by the two different types of oxidation, the denaturation of hemoglobin on the one hand, and the oxidation of heme iron on the other. This is particularly so since both effects can be produced by certain oxidant drugs. However, clinical manifestations usually depend on an underlying metabolic defect, and any given individual will have but one abnormality. Either there is a hemolytic anemia due to a defect in aerobic metabolism or cyanosis due to impaired methemoglobin reduction and/or the formation of sulfhemoglobin.

The Luebering-Rapaport pathway bypasses the direct formation of 3PG from 1,3-DPG and permits the accumulation of 2,3-DPG. The apparent reason for the large amount of this compound found in the red cell (1 mole DPG/1 mole Hb) lies in its profound effect on the affinity of hemoglobin for oxygen. Not only is red cell DPG essential for maintaining the basal PO_2 at a level suitable for O_2 transport, but it also plays a regulatory role in O_2 transport (25). Regulation occurs in the following fashion: whenever O_2 supply to peripheral tissues is reduced, the proportion extracted from the blood in systemic capillaries increases. The increase in reduced hemoglobin within the red cell results in increased binding of DPG and stimulates glycolysis, perhaps through a pH change within the cell, resulting in an increase in total red cell DPG and ATP. The increased concentration of these ligands in turn produces a right shift in the O_2 dissociation curve, making more oxygen available at any given O_2 tension. When available O_2 is increased above normal by acidosis (Bohr effect), red cell

9

glycolysis is reduced and the DPG level falls to a level just sufficient to normalize the in vivo P_{50} if sufficient time is allowed for equilibrium (T 1/2 about 8 hours). The converse occurs with alkalosis. Thus the red cell has an inbuilt mechanism low in energy cost which is capable of regulating O_2 transport, in both hypoxic states and acid-base imbalance.

D. Red Cell Breakdown

The normal red cell has a finite life-span in circulation of 120 + 20 days. As the cell becomes older, certain glycolytic enzymes decrease in activity, membrane is lost, the mean cell hemoglobin concentration increases, and cell pliability decreases. When these changes have reached a critical point, the red cell is no longer able to traverse the microvasculature and is phagocytized by the reticuloendothelial tissue (RE).

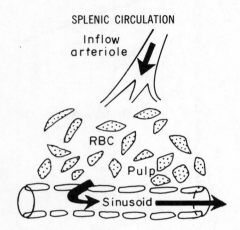

SPLENIC CIRCULATION

While all RE cells participate in the destruction of senescent red cells, those in the spleen are so situated anatomically as to be the most sensitive detectors of a red cell abnormality. Blood enters the reticular mesh-work of the splenic red cell pulp through terminal arterial branches. Blood flow is slow and the volume of plasma is reduced, exposing the red cell to the phagocytic action of RE cells (5). Intact red cells return to circulation via the venous sinusoids, where cell pliability is tested by the small sinusoidal orifices (3-5 μ). There, abnormal particles are removed along with some cell membrane. The quality control which the spleen exerts on the circulating red cell mass is evident from the increase in circulating abnormal forms after splenectomy, including nuclear remnants (Howell-Jolly bodies), denatured hemoglobin inclusions (Heinz bodies), siderocytes and misshapen or fragmented cells (p. 58).

RETICULOENDOTHELIAL CATABOLISM OF THE RED CELL

| Extravascular Destruction |

A phago-cytized red cell is attacked by the lysosomes of the RE cell. The hemoglobin molecule is disassembled, its iron returned to plasma transferrin for use by the erythroid marrow, and its amino acids redirected into the body protein pool (26). The protoporphyrin ring is broken at the alpha methene bridge by a

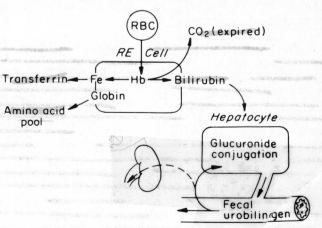

heme oxidase enzyme (27), and the alpha carbon is exhaled as carbon monoxide (28). The opened tetrapyrrole (bilirubin) is carried by plasma albumin to the liver where it is conjugated to glucuronide and excreted in the bile (29). Both unconjugated (prehepatic) and conjugated (post-hepatic) bilirubin are present in the plasma. They can be differentiated by the rate of reaction with diazo dye; unconjugated reacts slowly (indirected reacting) while the conjugated form reacts rapidly (direct reacting). The bilirubin glucuronide excreted into the gut is further converted through bacterial action to urobilinogen (stercobilinogen). Most of this is recovered in the stool, while a small amount of resorbed urobilinogen appears in the urine.

Intravascular erythrocyte breakdown represents an ancillary pathway of pigment catabolism, normally accounting for less than 10% of red cell destruction. Hemoglobin released directly into the blood stream undergoes dissociation into alpha-beta dimers which are quickly bound to the plasma globulin, haptoglobin (30). Formation of the HpHb complex prevents the renal excretion of plasma hemoglobin and stabilizes the heme-globin bond.

| Intravascular Destruction |

The complex is removed from circulation by hepatocyte uptake (31) and is processed within that cell in a fashion similar to that described for whole red cell catabolism. Because haptoglobin is removed as the HpHb complex, its level in plasma falls with hemolysis. Once plasma haptoglobin is depleted, unbound hemoglobin dimers are rapidly filtered by the renal glomerulus, only to be resorbed by renal tubular cells, and converted to hemosiderin. As much as 5 gm per day of filtered hemoglobin may be so processed without exceeding the tubular uptake capacity. Above that level, free hemoglobin and met-hemoglobin appear in the urine.

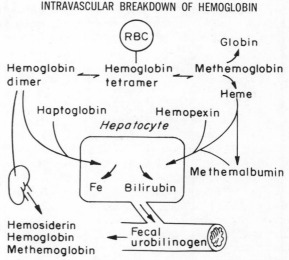

INTRAVASCULAR BREAKDOWN OF HEMOGLOBIN

Later, when the tubular cells are desquamated into the urine, their hemosiderin granules give indication of prior hemoglobinemia. Thus, renal processing of filtered hemoglobin may result in the excretion of hemosiderin alone, hemosiderin and hemoglobin, or hemoglobin alone if hemolysis is acute and massive.

Hemoglobin which is neither bound by haptoglobin nor processed by the *Hemopexin* kidneys is oxidized to methemoglobin, whereupon heme groups are released and taken up by another transport protein, hemopexin (32). This heme-hemopexin complex is cleared from circulation by the hepatocyte and catabolized. Heme groups in excess of the hemopexin-binding capacity combine with albumin to form methemalbumin and are held by this protein until additional hemopexin becomes available to shuttle the heme to the hepatocyte.

Normally the hemoglobin-binding capacity of plasma haptoglobin is 50-200 mg%, and that of hemopexin is 50-100 mg%. The combined depletion of haptoglobin and hemopexin and the presence of methemalbuminemia and hemosiderinuria is seen not only with hemolytic anemia but also with intramarrow destruction of red cell precursors (ineffective erythropoiesis). Hemopexin depletion and methemalbumin formation without hemosiderinuria is said to occur with bleeding into the tissues, as for example, intra-abdominal bleeding in ectopic pregnancy.

II. QUANTITATIVE ASPECTS OF ERYTHROPOIESIS

A. Erythrokinetics

The erythron may be arbitrarily divided into a fixed portion of normoblasts and reticulocytes residing within the marrow, and a circulating portion of reticulocytes and adult red cells. The relative number of these cell populations and the time spent at each phase of development is shown in the accompanying table. Because of the slow turnover of circulating red cells (1% per day), a relatively small erythroid marrow is able to sustain a large circulating red cell mass in the normal subject under basal conditions.

CELL TYPE	TIME SPAN (DAYS)	CELL NUMBER (10^9/kg)
Nucleated RBC	4	4.5
Marrow reticulocytes	2.5	7.5
Blood reticulocytes	1	3
Adult RBC	120	300
	CIRCULATING MASS	DAILY TURNOVER (70 kg man)
Red Cells	2000 ml	17 ml
Hemoglobin	660 gm	5.7 gm
Porphyrin pigment	23 gm	190 mg
Iron	2.2 gm	18 mg

In disease, the size of the erythron may be greatly altered. With decreased stimulation, the erythroid marrow activity can decrease to less than 1/3 its basal size with a corresponding fall in circulating red cells. Likewise, with an impairment in proliferation (damage to the stem cell pool), the mass of both fixed and circulating erythroid cells will decrease. On the other hand, with maturation disorders (ineffective erythropoiesis) or when there is increased destruction of circulating red cells, erythrocyte precursors are increased under the stimulus of erythropoietin while the circulating red cell mass is reduced through the rapid destruction of developing or mature erythrocytes. Changes in the erythroid marrow and circulating red cell mass as well as the characteristic red cell life-span for each situation are shown diagrammatically in the figure on the next page.

MARROW/CIRCULATING RED CELL RELATIONSHIPS IN
DISTURBANCES OF THE ERYTHRON

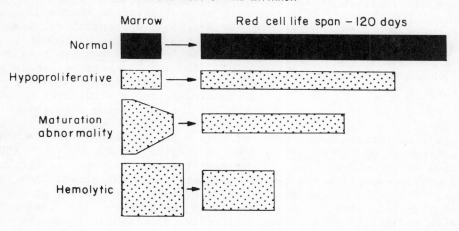

The various points at which quantitative measurements of red cell turnover may be made are illustrated in the accompanying figure. These are measurements of total erythropoiesis (reflecting the degree of proliferation of the erythroid marrow), effective erythropoiesis (representing only that portion of erythropoiesis which leads to circulating cells), total hemoglobin catabolism (derived from both marrow and circulating red cell breakdown), and circulating red cell breakdown.

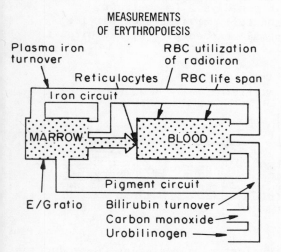

The clinical approach to anemia places major emphasis on quantitative measurements of erythropoiesis. This requires the conversion of individual measurements of production and destruction to a common expression which permits comparison, generally an index of production. Destruction measurements are converted with the assumption that the individual is in red cell equilibrium, i.e. production equals destruction (p. 68). The index may be then compared to normal basal red cell production in that individual. Total or effective erythropoiesis is characterized as a fraction or multiple of 1 (basal production) and the patient's marrow response described in the context of the response to anemia expected of a normal marrow.

$$\frac{N^o \text{ of Erythroid}}{\text{granulocytic cell in B/M aspirate}} = E/G.$$

PRODUCTION MEASUREMENTS

I. Effective erythropoiesis
   Reticulocyte index
   Red cell iron turnover
II. Total erythropoiesis
   Erythrocyte/granulocyte ratio
   Erythron iron turnover

Circulating reticulo count!

Red Cell Production

Red cell production may be quantified in several ways. The total proliferative status of the erythroid marrow is evaluated by comparing the number of erythroid to granulocytic cells in the marrow aspirate (E/G ratio). The most convenient laboratory test for evaluating effective red cell production is the circulating reticulocyte count corrected for maturation time (p. 60).

A more quantitative measurement of both total and effective erythropoiesis is provided by the erythron iron turnover employing radioiron. About 80% of the iron carried by transferrin goes to the erythron, and the exact distribution (erythron versus non-erythron) can be calculated from the plasma iron level and plasmatocrit (33). In the absence of iron deficiency the amount of erythron iron uptake (EIT) is directly proportional to the number of developing erythroid cells and thus total erythropoiesis. Effective erythropoiesis may be evaluated by measuring the proportion of injected radioiron appearing in the red cell mass (per cent utilization) (34). In combination with *in vivo* counting it is possible to characterize the major patterns of abnormal erythropoiesis. In the normal individual, radioiron uptake by the marrow is rapid and redelivery to circulation (red cell activity) takes place over the next ten days. In contrast, abnormalities in proliferation, maturation and cell survival show varying patterns of liver and spleen uptake and abnormal reappearance of radioiron in blood.

FERROKINETIC PROFILES

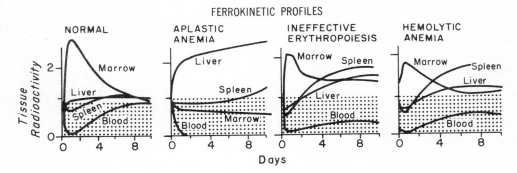

Red Cell Destruction

Red cell destruction is evaluated by measuring CO production (28), bilirubin turnover (35), fecal urobilinogen (36) and red cell life span (p. 69). The first three measure the total amount of hemoglobin pigment being catabolized regardless of whether it is derived from the breakdown of circulating red cells or from ineffective erythropoiesis. These procedures are not in general use and their results are not highly quantitative, particularly at low levels of erythropoiesis. Red cell life span measurements reflect the turnover of circulating red cells and have more clinical utility. However, this

DESTRUCTION MEASUREMENTS

I. Effective (circulating red cell)
   Cr^{51} survival
   DFP^{32} survival
II. Total red cell catabolism
   Fecal urobilinogen
   Exhaled carbon monoxide
   Bilirubin turnover

measurement does not evaluate intramarrow destruction and it is insensitive to red cell destruction occurring shortly after their entrance into circulation.

B. Substrates for Erythropoiesis

Deficiency of several dietary substances can cause anemia: iron, folate, B$_{12}$, protein and a miscellaneous group (copper, pyridoxine, vitamin E, etc.) whose roles in the production of anemia in man are less well defined. Uncomplicated protein deficiency produces a moderate decrease in hemoglobin concentration and red cell mass (20-30%), but this decrease is in keeping with the depletion of other body tissues (37). Thus, in a physiologic sense, the fall in hemoglobin associated with the protein deficiency cannot be considered an anemia, particularly since other body proteins can be mobilized for hemoglobin production if oxygen transport is suboptimal even in severe protein depletion (38).

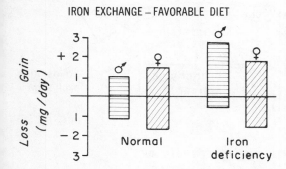

IRON EXCHANGE – FAVORABLE DIET

Iron is an essential part of the hemoglobin molecule, and any decrease in iron supply below the requirements of the erythroid marrow causes a proportionate decrease in hemoglobin synthesis. Most body iron exists as hemoglobin in the circulating red cell mass or is stored as ferritin and hemosiderin in RE and parenchymal tissues. Long-term iron balance is determined by the absorptive capacity as compared to growth requirements and excretory losses. The narrow margin between the amount of iron available for absorption and requirements in infants and the adult female largely accounts for the world-wide prevalence of iron deficiency, estimated at 500 million people. External iron exchange, the amount of iron required from the diet to replace losses, averages about 10% of the body iron content a year in the male and 15% in menstruating females, equivalent to 0.9 and 1.3 mg daily respectively (39). Dietary iron content is closely related to total caloric intake (approximately 6 mg/1000 calories). In the U.S. male, iron intake amounts to about 15 mg/day with 6% absorption, whereas in the average female daily intake is 11 mg with 12% absorption. An iron-deficient subject can increase iron absorption to about 20% of the iron present in a meat-containing diet, but only 5-10% in a vegetarian diet (40).

Iron Metabolism

BODY IRON CONTENT

	80 kg ♂	65 kg ♀
Erythron iron	2400	1700
Iron stores	1000 ± 200	300 ± 300
Myoglobin/ tissue iron	160	120
Transferrin iron	6	4

Since day to day absorption from diet is limited, body iron stores assume importance in meeting any immediate need for more iron such as during regeneration of red cells after blood loss. The individual's iron stores reflect the state of his external iron exchange over many years. Males, with a more favorable balance, are able to accrue stores of about 1000 mg. Females have an additional menstrual loss so their average stores amount to about 300 mg, with about 1/3 of the female population having virtually no iron stores (41). In the pregnant female, iron stores are so frequently inadequate that medicinal iron must be routinely prescribed. An equally adverse situation is found in infancy, where the routine fortification of milk and milk supplements with iron is recommended (42).

Internal iron exchange is largely concerned with red cell production. Ordinarily about 80% of iron passing through the plasma transferrin pool is derived from broken down red cells and marrow. As long as transferrin saturation is maintained between 20 and 60% and erythroid requirements for iron are not greatly increased, internal iron metabolism is adequate. In event of blood loss, up to 40 mg of iron per day may be mobilized for red cell production in the individual with iron stores of 500-1000 mg.

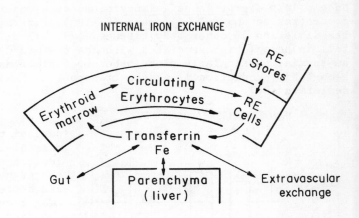

INTERNAL IRON EXCHANGE

SEQUENTIAL CHANGES IN THE DEVELOPMENT OF IRON DEFICIENCY

	Normal	Iron Depletion	Iron Deficient Erythropoiesis	Iron Deficiency Anemia
Iron Stores →				
Erythron Iron →				
RE Marrow Fe	2-3 +	0-1 +	0	0
Transferrin IBC (µg/100 ml)	330 ± 30	360	390	410
Plasma ferritin (µg/ml)	100 ± 60	20	10	< 10
Iron absorption (%)	5-10	10-15	10-20	10-20
Plasma iron (µg/100 ml);	115 ± 50	115	< 60	< 40
Transferrin saturation (%)	35 ± 15	30	< 15	< 10
Sideroblasts (%)	40-60	40-60	< 10	< 10
RBC Protoporphyrin (µg/100 ml RBC)	30	30	100	200
Erythrocytes	Normal	Normal	Normal	Microcytic/ Hypochromic

16

In the face of a negative iron balance, iron stores are mobilized first and then functional body iron is progressively depleted. Three stages of iron deficiency may be recognized: 1) Iron depletion where the hemosiderin content of the RE cells in the marrow aspirate is decreased or absent. Coincident with a decrease in these stores, mucosal absorption of iron increases, plasma transferrin level increases, and the plasma ferritin level falls. 2) Iron-deficient erythropoiesis where there is not only exhaustion of iron stores but also a fall in plasma iron below 30 mg%, and the transferrin saturation drops to less than 15% accompanied by an increase in red cell protoporphyrin. The decreased iron supply limits hemoglobin synthesis although there may be no recognizable anemia at the time. 3) Iron deficiency anemia where in addition to the other abnormalities mentioned, there is a demonstrable anemia which eventually is characterized by a decrease in red cell volume and hemoglobin concentration (microcytosis and hypochromia).

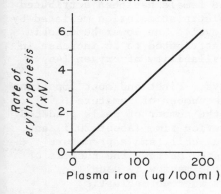

LIMITATION OF ERYTHROPOIESIS
BY PLASMA IRON LEVEL

The term relative iron deficient erythropoiesis is applied to situations where iron supply is adequate for basal erythropoiesis but inadequate for increased erythron requirements. While the adequacy of iron supply can be estimated from the saturation of transferrin in low output states (p. 63), it is difficult to use this parameter when marrow needs are increased by increased red cell production. This is particularly relevant to the patient with a compensated hemolytic process when a superimposed inflammatory state reduces a high normal plasma iron to a low normal level. Since iron supply is then insufficient to sustain the high rate of erythropoiesis, anemia results. In determining the adequacy of iron supply in such a setting, the protoporphyrin concentration of the circulating red cells is especially useful (43). This measurement directly reflects the balance between iron supply and the need for hemoglobin synthesis within individual cells (p. 64).

Inflammation interferes with iron exchange by blocking the release of catabolized red cell iron from RE cells. At the same time red cell life span is shortened, thereby increasing erythron iron requirements. The iron blockade plus hemolysis render iron supply insufficient to meet marrow needs. Transferrin saturation falls to less that 20% and protoporphyrin increases in the red cells. Eventually red cells become slightly hypochromic and microcytic. Iron deficient erythropoiesis due to inflammation is therefore similar to true iron deficiency in that plasma iron is inadequate to support the increase required for erythropoiesis; it differs, however, by the continued presence of hemosiderin within the RE cell of the marrow.

RE CELL IRON BLOCKADE

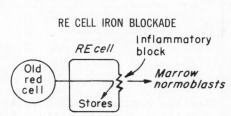

C. Stimulated Erythropoiesis

Red cell production is regulated by the output of erythropoietin from the kidney; an increase in erythropoiesis is
dependent upon an increase in this stimulating hormone (44).

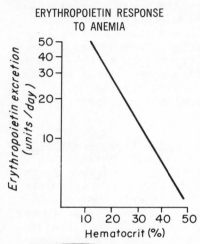

ERYTHROPOIETIN RESPONSE
TO ANEMIA

Bioassay methods for erythropoietin are not
sufficiently sensitive to detect plasma levels in
the normal subject, but measurable amounts are
demonstrated by urinary assay. The excretion of
erythropoietin changes logarithmically in relation
to the hemoglobin concentration of the blood (45).
The renal sensor mechanism also responds to changes
in arterial O_2 saturation and hemoglobin affinity
for O_2. Various hormones also affect erythropoietin production; for example, the response curve
is shifted to the left with deficiencies of
testosterone, glucocorticoids, and thyroxin. The
lower hemoglobin in the female has been attributed
to decreased erythropoietin stimulation mediated by
a lower testosterone level. The lower hemoglobin
of childhood has been attributed to an increase in
DPG which increases availability of oxygen (46).

Erythropoietin acts on the marrow in several ways. First and most important
is its effect on committed stem cells to increase the number of immature
erythroid cells undergoing maturation and therefore the number of cells produced.
Other effects include a modest decrease in the maturation time (about 20%), an
increase in hemoglobin synthesis within the individual cell, and a premature
release of marrow reticulocytes (47). In the stimulated marrow, the nucleus of
the developing normoblasts is somewhat enlarged and the marrow is usually
described as macronormoblastic.
Provided the supply of iron is optimal,
red cells under the influence of
increased erythropoietin have a greater
than normal amount of hemoglobin, but a
slightly decreased hemoglobin concentration. The basal marrow reticulocyte
maturation time of about 3 days (as
measured by radioiron) becomes
progressively shortened as the erythropoietin level increases. This really
represents a premature release of marrow
reticulocytes as reflected in the
appearance of basophilic macroreticulo-
cytes in the blood smear. Such "shift"
cells have a diameter about 25% greater
than that of surrounding cells (48).

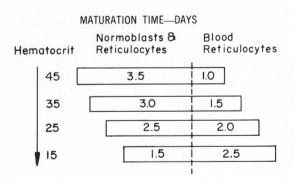

MATURATION TIME—DAYS

Hematocrit	Normoblasts & Reticulocytes	Blood Reticulocytes
45	3.5	1.0
35	3.0	1.5
25	2.5	2.0
15	1.5	2.5

When the hematocrit is normal, less than 5% of all reticulocytes have the
characteristics of shift cells. As the hematocrit falls, this percentage

increases exponentially. The absolute number of shift cells on a blood smear is a function not only of the degree of erythropoietin stimulation but also of the total number of reticulocytes present. The accompanying figure shows shift cells from a normal individual exposed to the hypoxia of high altitude (a), and from patients with megaloblastic (b), hemolytic (c), and iron deficiency anemias (d). Understanding and allowing for shift is essential in the use of the reticulocyte count as a measure of erythropoiesis (p. 59).

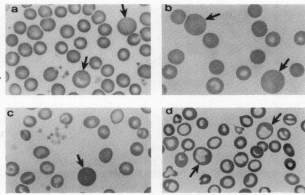

SHIFT CELLS

Response to hypoxia or anemia has a certain lag time. While an increase in erythropoietin is demonstrable within about 6 hours, and a shift in reticulocytes appears within 1 or 2 days, 4 to 6 days are required for full response of the erythroid marrow and 6 to 8 days for a maximum reticulocyte response. Much longer time is required for a significant increase in the red cell mass. With longstanding anemia, the erythroid marrow expands into the long bones and sometimes into extramedullary sites. With severe congenital anemias, the marrow cavity of developing bones becomes large enough to produce visible deformities, particularly evident in the skull (frontal bossing, tower skull, and protruding maxillae.)

The full capacity of the erythroid marrow for red cell production is only apparent when there is maximal erythropoietin stimulation and an unlimited supply of iron. Under

> Maximal Red
> Cell Production

such circumstances red cell production can increase within one week to 5 times normal. With continued stimulation the marrow gradually extends into new bony areas, and production rates exceeding 8 times normal may be achieved. Submaximal red cell production is usually not the result of impaired erythropoietin production but rather depends on the availability of iron. Only with a hemolytic process where there is increased red cell catabolism will iron supply be maximal. By contrast, the average adult male with iron stores of about 1000 mg and a hemoglobin decreased by bleeding to 12 gm%, mobilizes only about 20 mg of iron from his reserves per day and therefore increases red cell production to no more than twice normal. If bleeding is severe enough to reduce the hemoglobin to 7 gm%, approximately 30-40 mg of storage iron can be mobilized and erythropoiesis increases to about 2.5 times normal. The actual rate achieved in blood loss anemia is therefore dependent on the size of the pre-existing iron stores. The individual without iron stores can increase production by no more than a tenth of normal since he is limited by the 1-3 mg of extra iron which can be derived from diet. Sustained production at about 3 times normal and temporary production at even higher levels may be achieved when oral or parenteral iron is provided in large amounts (49,50).

III. O$_2$ TRANSPORT

A. Blood Volume and Flow

The circulating blood is contained within a vascular container composed of large vessels which function as conduits and a capillary interface for exchange between the blood and interstitial fluids. Arteries contain about 20%, capillaries 10%, and veins 70% of the total volume. Thus, the veins represent the major storage area for blood. Volume is measured by the dilution of intravenously injected materials (p. 65). The most convenient expression of blood volume is ml/kg, but the most accurate expression is based on surface area or lean body mass (51). All reference points have limitations when applied to the individual, for blood volume is affected by changes in body composition, physical activity, and environmental factors which affect metabolic rate (52). For example, when blood volume is expressed on a per kilogram basis, the amount of fat is important because it is relatively avascular. A variety of physiologic and pathologic factors determine the appropriate blood volume for an individual. Physical conditioning and hypermetabolism increase volume by 10 to 30%, the opposite is true with hypometabolism. Simple bed rest decreases volume by about 10% in 1 or 2 weeks.

Normal Blood Volume

Warm weather is associated with cutaneous vasodilatation and an increase in total volume. Extreme weight loss increases blood volume per kilo due to the greater preservation of blood as compared with other body tissues. Distortion of a portion of the vascular bed may result in a corresponding change in volume; thus, an increase of as much as 50% may be seen with caval obstruction or in patients with the block in the microvasculature produced by macroglobulinemia or sickle cell anemia.

NORMAL BLOOD VOLUME
(ml/kg)

	♂	♀
Total	70	65
Red cell mass	30	25
Plasma volume	40	40

Regulation of Blood Volume

The physiologic implications of the blood volume are largely related to venous blood return to the heart. Cardiac output is decreased by a reduction in venous return, while an increased return increases output. It is primarily the plasma volume which changes in accord the subject's body composition, metabolic needs, and vascular container so as to optimize cardiac output. Plasma volume has two points of regulation: 1) internal regulation which is achieved at the capillary membrane by an exchange with extravascular fluid according to the principles defined in Starling's law. Thus, plasma volume may drop when the pressure rises in the microvasculature (catecholamines) or plasma oncotic pressure falls (hypoalbuminemia). 2) external regulation which is accomplished by volume

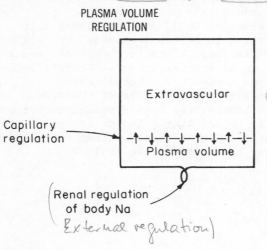

PLASMA VOLUME REGULATION

Extravascular

Capillary regulation

Plasma volume

Renal regulation of body Na

(External regulation)

20

receptors determining the renal excretion of sodium. If blood volume is lost through hemorrhage or extravascular fluid shift, sodium is retained by the kidney until plasma volume is repleted.

Regulation of blood volume by changes in total extracellular fluid is a slow adjustment, and the individual would be in serious difficulty if the vascular system could not accommodate through changes in vasomotor tone. Pressure regulation of the venous blood reservoir by the sympathetic nervous system and catecholamines make it possible for normal individuals to maintain an adequate circulation in the face of a sudden decrease or removal of up to 20% of total blood volume. At the same time, vasomotor regulation can fluctuate spontaneously from minute to minute and is affected by emotions and drugs. Thus, clinical manifestations of circulatory insufficiency must be interpreted in relation to both volume and vasomotor components. Moderate hypovolemia may be tolerated without pulse or blood pressure changes under normal circumstances, but may cause orthostatic hypotension and syncope when there is cutaneous vaso-dilatation secondary to heat or with vasodepressor drugs. The patient with hypovolemia due to gastrointestinal bleeding may have few symptoms until he sees the tarry stool when the emotional reaction may produce vasodilatation and syncope.

Total blood volume is determined by independent regulating mechanisms for red cell mass and plasma volume. When changes in plasma volume are imposed, the erythron seeks to maintain an appropriate hemoglobin concentration. Thus, the chronic enlargement of blood volume with cardiac failure or the decrease in volume associated with chronic salt depletion of Addison's disease results in a proportionate change in red cell mass. The overriding regulatory consideration for the erythron is the maintenance of O_2 transport. Changes in the red cell mass appear to evoke changes in plasma volume designed to maintain optimal blood flow. Anemia is associated with an increase in plasma volume so as to maintain a nearly normal total volume. With an increase in the red cell mass, plasma volume is maintained at normal levels, probably the best compromise between the hypervolemic and viscosity problems imposed by polycythemia.

TISSUE OXYGEN SUPPLY
AND ITS REGULATION

O_2 Transport

The purpose of the red cell is to mediate oxygen transport between lung and peripheral tissues. As previously discussed, the red cell influences O_2 transport in two ways, first by the concentration of hemoglobin in the blood which determines the O_2 carrying capacity, and second by the regulation of the hemoglobin affinity for O_2 which determines the amount of O_2 released at

21

any given O_2 tension. Other essential components in the O_2 transport system are shown in the accompanying figure (53). Ventilation plays two roles: It is responsible on the one hand for O_2 loading of red cells and on the other for maintenance of acid-base balance through the regulation of CO_2 (which in itself influences the availability of oxygen through the Bohr effect). The heart and cardiovascular system determine the amount of blood pumped per unit time to the tissues. The distribution of this flow is regulated locally by the autonomic nervous system. These components must function together so that the composite tissue requirements for oxygen are met.

Each supply mechanism is under a different regulation. Ventilation responds to changes in pH and CO_2 as well as to hypoxia. Cardiac output responds to the amount of blood entering the heart, and this is principally regulated by the metabolism of peripheral tissues as it affects resistance in the microvasculature. The erythron responds to changes in hemoglobin concentration, arterial O_2 saturation and hemoglobin affinity by altering the rate of erythropoiesis.

Since the O_2 requirements of the body must be met, a decreased capacity of any one component is corrected by an increased function of other components. More specifically, a decrease of arterial O_2 loading due to a lowered ambient O_2 tension or pulmonary disease, results in an increased ventilation, an increased hemoglobin concentration and a right shift in the O_2 dissociation curve due to an increase in 2,3-DPG. If increased ventilation is possible, alkalosis is produced which in time is corrected by an increased renal loss of body base. Decreased cardiac output is not associated with an increase in hemoglobin concentration, but rather with compensatory shunting of blood from areas of high flow to more critical tissues and a shift in the oxygen dissociation curve mediated by DPG. Moderate anemia is associated with a shift in the O_2 dissociation curve and blood shunting; at lower levels of hemoglobin concentration there is an increase in cardiac output as well and some hyperventilation. Increased tissue O_2 consumption as in thyrotoxicosis is almost entirely counterbalanced by an increased cardiac output. Since multiple defects may have additive consequences, it is important in dealing with anemia to recognize any impairment in the normal compensatory response.

Hypoxia is difficult to define in terms which are clinically useful. Symptoms are non-specific. The actual measurement of O_2 consumption means little, since the needs of the individual cannot be precisely predicted, and since a deficit in O_2 consumption rarely occurs. Mean venous oxygen tension probably comes closest to defining O_2 supply. In most mammalian species including man, the mean venous PO_2 is 40 mm Hg, and any decrease indicates either that there is shunting of blood from high to low flow areas (a reduction in O_2 reserve), or that the tissue pressure of O_2 in vital tissues is actually reduced (hypoxia). The clinical approach relies primarily on an analysis of the function of the individual components (ventilation, cardiac output, hemoglobin concentration, and O_2 saturation) with therapeutic efforts directed at any one which appears abnormal.

PART 2 CLINICAL APPROACH

I.   ANEMIA

A. Manifestations of Anemia

As the hemoglobin concentration falls below the physiologic norm for the individual, there is a proportionate decrease in maximal O_2 transport capacity (54). With mild anemia this may be reflected in a slight increase in dyspnea, palpitation, and sweating which ordinarily accompany exercise. With moderate anemia, these symptoms become more definite and are often associated with excessive fatigue. Severe anemia results in marked exertional and non-exertional dyspnea, pounding pulse (wide pulse pressure) associated with an increased cardiac output and decreased peripheral resistance, hypersensitivity to cold secondary to decreased skin blood flow, and loss of appetite with indigestion due to inadequate splanchnic O_2 supply (55). Generalized weakness, dizziness, and occasionally syncope may occur. Central nervous system symptoms include headache, insomnia, Cheyne-Stokes respiration during sleep, inability to concentrate, etc. While the relatively nonspecific symptoms described above may result from anemia alone, they are more easily provoked with abnormalitites of more than one link in the O_2 transport chain. Their presence at a hemoglobin of 10 gm% or more is more likely due to underlying disease affecting cardiopulmonary function or vasomotor regulation than anemia per se. Blood volume depletion may compromise blood flow in patients with anemia due to hemorrhage. The cumulative effects of anemia and local vascular disease are particularly important. Examples include coronary atherosclerosis producing angina or failure, peripheral vascular disease producing intermittent claudication, and cerebrovascular disease resulting in disorientation or impaired vasomotor regulation.

The presence of anemia is not accurately detected on physical examination. The patient's skin color is as much dependent on skin thickness, blood distribution and melanin pigmentation as on hemoglobin concentration. The myxedematous or nephrotic patient is pale because the blood in the skin is particularly obscured by subcutaneous fluid, whereas the patient with atrophic skin (Cushing's disease) or with cutaneous vasodilatation may have normal color despite a decreased red cell mass. The best areas for evaluating hemoglobin concentration are the conjunctivae and mucous membranes, since epidermal thickness is more uniform and thermal effects on blood content are minimized. Chronic anemia of sufficient severity to increase cardiac output is usually associated with an increase in stroke volume; the presence of tachycardia suggests volume depletion, heart disease, or increased tissue O_2 requirements (inflammation).

B. Detection of Anemia

Evaluation of the hemoglobin concentration in a particular individual requires careful consideration of any environmental or personal factors which may modify the hemoglobin concentration. For example, altitude has a predictable effect (p. 47). Any other condition which produces arterial O_2 desaturation may increase hemoglobin concentration, i.e. pulmonary disease. A distinction is therefore made <u>between laboratory and physiologic anemia</u>. Laboratory anemia is based on population criteria with the realization of its limits when applied to the individual. <u>Physiologic anemia is defined as the presence of an inappropriately low hemoglobin</u> for the individual in the context of all components of O_2 supply and demand.

Definition of Anemia

Anemia is usually defined in terms of the hemoglobin concentration. Arbitrary hemoglobin values for the general population and the limit below which anemia is likely to be present are shown in the accompanying table. However, these figures provide a general laboratory definition of anemia and may not be appropriate for the individual. Many people have a hemoglobin concentration which is physiologically normal for them, but which is defined by comparison with general population data, as anemia. Still other individuals will have a hemoglobin level physiologically subnormal for them, even though it falls within the range considered normal for the general population. Indeed, the

	MEAN NORMAL VALUES	
AGE	HEMOGLOBIN	HEMATOCRIT
	g/100 ml	%
Birth	17.0	50
1 to 3 months	14.0	42
3 months to 5 years	12.0	36
6 to 10 years	12.0	37
11 to 15 years	13.0	39
Adult male	15.0	47
Menstruating female	13.5	41
Pregnancy (last trimester)	12.0	37

number of adult females erroneously classified as normal by standard criteria is probably as great as the number of females correctly identified as having anemia (56). The accompanying figure shows the probability of anemia in: 1) a population of women whose mean normal hemoglobin is <u>13.5 gm% + 1 gm%</u> and with an assumed 10% prevalence of anemia; and 2) 2) a population of men with a mean normal hemoglobin of <u>15 gm% + 1 gm%</u> with an assumed 4% prevalence of anemia. This figure demonstrates that the recognition of mild anemia is inexact when based on hemoglobin concentration alone.

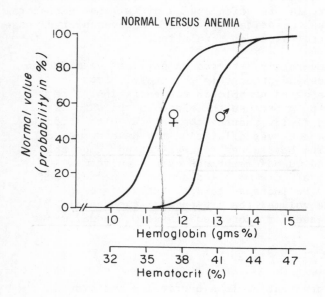

NORMAL VERSUS ANEMIA

If one were only concerned about the adequacy of O_2 transport, the recognition of mild anemia would be of little consequence. However, anemia usually provides a signal of underlying disease, such as bleeding neoplasm, infection, renal failure, or endocrinopathy. Thus, early recognition of mild anemia may be very important. Since the most frequent general cause of mild anemia is iron deficient erythropoiesis, physiologic anemia may be identified by demonstrating iron deficiency while the hemoglobin concentration is still within "normal limits." This early recognition permits a further search for the cause, i.e. bleeding or inflammation.

C. General Therapeutic Considerations

In the severely anemic patient with hypoxic symptoms (often involving the central nervous system), O_2 administration by nasal catheter or mask is usually desirable. Such a procedure can provide the severely anemic patient with two to three volumes percent of additional O_2 in the plasma and thereby increase O_2 transport by 25 to 50%. Blood transfusion may be employed to produce a rapid increase in hemoglobin and thereby O_2 carrying capacity. Sufficient red cells should be administered to relieve the patient's hypoxia. Patients who are free of cardiovascular disease are quite comfortable with a chronic anemia of 7 gm% and do not require transfusion at that level. When the presence of symptoms in the patient with chronic anemia indicates the need for transfusion, packed red cells are employed. It is often desirable to minimize the problem of volume overload by administering a potent diuretic such as furosemide or by removing an equivalent volume of the patient's blood, before packed cells are administered. Whole blood transfusion is indicated when both hemoglobin concentration and total blood volume are decreased sufficient to represent a danger to the patient.

| Blood Transfusion |

The presence of syncope, hypotension and tachycardia raises the question of hypovolemia and requires the usual workup for shock. Clinical evaluation of the blood volume begins with an examination of the venous system and measurement of intravascular pressure. Some indication of volume change is obtained at the bedside by the size and filling of neck veins, provided the patient is flat in bed and breathing easily. The jugular vein is usually visible 1 cm above the lower margin of the sterno-cleidomastoid muscle. The adequacy of venous return can also be assessed by peripheral or better by central venous pressure measurements. If circulation appears adequate in the recumbent position, the patient should be examined standing. Since this position causes pooling of about 500 ml of blood in the lower extremities of adults, the ability to stand without a significant drop in arterial pressure (less than 20 mm Hg) indicates a volume reserve of at least 500 ml. While changes in pulse rate and in arterial and venous pressures may be due to hypovolemia, it must be appreciated that similar effects are produced by independent changes in vascular tone, cardiac output, and peripheral tissue O_2 requirements.

| Hypovolemia |

Direct blood volume measurement may be used in some situations (p. 65). When well-performed, these procedures carry a technical error of only about 5%. However, the difficulty of estimating the physiologic norm of a given individual

25

is a far greater obstacle. Furthermore, the significance of any volume change depends on the extent to which the patient can accommodate. When there is impaired vascular control or myocardial damage, changes of clinical significance may be too small to evaluate by direct measurement. In such situations, monitoring the venous pressure is a more useful approach, because venous return is critical to cardiac output. Volume measurements are sometimes helpful in differentiating between hypovolemia and vascular dysfunction, and sequential measurements may assist in managing the seriously ill patient.

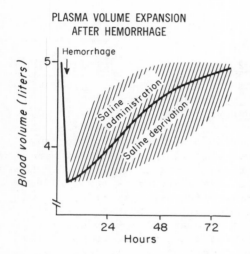

PLASMA VOLUME EXPANSION
AFTER HEMORRHAGE

The most common cause of hypovolemia is bleeding (accompanying trauma, operative procedures where blood replacement is inadequate, hemorrhage from the GI tract). The amount of bleeding with trauma is often underestimated; when a patient has three or more fractures, the average early blood loss is approximately 2000 ml, and continued bleeding may occur during the first week (57,58). Internal bleeding may be very difficult to recognize until the plasma volume reexpands and the hematocrit falls (59). The rate at which this occurs is variable since it depends on the intake of water and sodium (60). The first step in treatment of the bleeding patient is therefore administration of parenteral saline solution. Initial volume replacement carries very little likelihood of overload. Either whole blood or plasma volume expanders may be employed for more long-lasting effects, and their selection depends on the patient's hemoglobin concentration. Expanders may be used when the hemoglobin is over 10 gm%, although with continued bleeding, the hemoglobin soon falls below that level. When hemoglobin is less than 10 gm%, whole blood is desirable. In shock, re-establishment of adequate volume to sustain circulation takes precedence over hemoglobin replacement. With massive bleeding and massive transfusion, additional consideration must be given to the maintenance of hemostasis. The critical hemostatic component is the platelet, and platelet or fresh blood administration should be undertaken when the count falls below 50,000/mm^3.

Other components of O_2 transport must be examined in the chronically anemic patient where symptoms of hypoxia seem disproportionate to the degree of anemia. Anemia may preclude the development of cyanosis, since approximately 5 gm% of

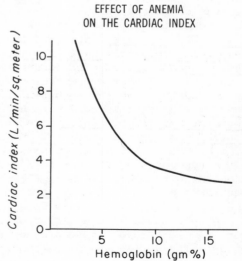

EFFECT OF ANEMIA
ON THE CARDIAC INDEX

26

reduced hemoglobin are required in order to recognize cyanosis. When pulmonary disease is suspected, arterial blood should be drawn for blood gas determinations and O_2 administered until the results are available. Cardiac status is evaluated by searching for the usual signs of heart disease, particularly cardiac enlargement and evidence of pulmonary congestion. Once the hemoglobin level falls below 7 or 8 gm, cardiac output must increase appreciably to maintain an adequate supply of O_2. Inadequate cardiac response is suggested by an absence of hyperactive heart sounds and systolic murmurs, lack of bounding pulse or by the presence of tachycardia (for chronic anemia per se does not produce tachycardia). Tissue O_2 requirements may be critical in the anemic patient, and are frequently increased by inflammation.

D. Diagnostic Approach to Anemia

INCIDENCE OF DIFFERENT ANEMIAS

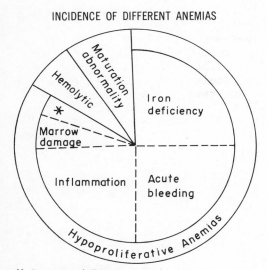

* Deceased Erythropoietin

The physician must first decide on the basis of the hemoglobin concentration and general information obtained in the history and physical examination, whether anemia is present and whether it can be readily explained or needs further study. While most anemias are associated with inadequate proliferation of the erythroid marrow (see figure), hemolytic and maturation abnormalities requiring specific therapy must be recognized. A systematic approach is therefore adopted in order to delineate the nature of the anemia in each patient. A physiologic classification is shown in the branching format on the following page. By applying simple laboratory tests, anemia may be classified on the basis of its cause, as a hemolytic or hypoproliferative state or as the result of a maturation abnormality. This classification is made by evaluation of the blood smear, red cell indices and and reticulocyte count. Further separation into subcategories is possible through additional laboratory tests.

Hemolytic anemia is recognized primarily by a high reticulocyte count. This is actually a measurement of effective red cell production, but there is no convenient or reliable way to quantify red cell destruction. Fortunately, red cell production and destruction are usually of similar magnitude (i.e., they have reached an equilibrium). Proper use of the reticulocyte count involves its conversion to an index which reflects the rate of red cell production. The "raw reticulocyte count" relates the number of reticulocytes to the number of red cells in circulation (percent retics). An initial correction is required to convert this figure to an absolute quantity, and a second correction for the effect of erythropoietin on reticulocyte release from the marrow (p. 18). The reticulocyte index, derived from this double correction, reflects the rate of red

| Initial |
| Laboratory |
| Approach |

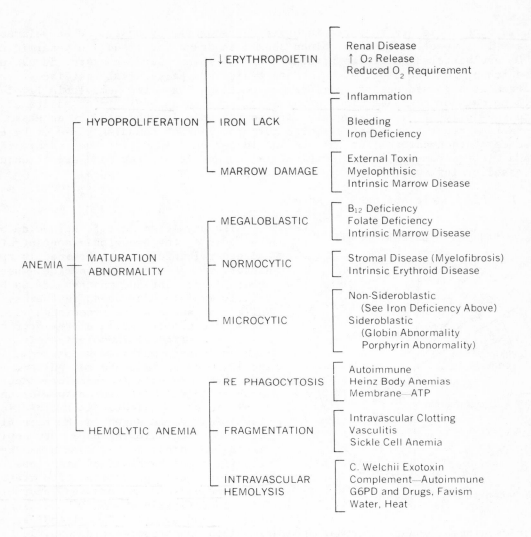

ANEMIA
- HYPOPROLIFERATION
  - ↓ ERYTHROPOIETIN
    - Renal Disease
    - ↑ O₂ Release
    - Reduced O₂ Requirement
  - IRON LACK
    - Inflammation
    - Bleeding
    - Iron Deficiency
  - MARROW DAMAGE
    - External Toxin
    - Myelophthisic
    - Intrinsic Marrow Disease
- MATURATION ABNORMALITY
  - MEGALOBLASTIC
    - B₁₂ Deficiency
    - Folate Deficiency
    - Intrinsic Marrow Disease
  - NORMOCYTIC
    - Stromal Disease (Myelofibrosis)
    - Intrinsic Erythroid Disease
  - MICROCYTIC
    - Non-Sideroblastic (See Iron Deficiency Above)
    - Sideroblastic (Globin Abnormality Porphyrin Abnormality)
- HEMOLYTIC ANEMIA
  - RE PHAGOCYTOSIS
    - Autoimmune
    - Heinz Body Anemias
    - Membrane—ATP
  - FRAGMENTATION
    - Intravascular Clotting
    - Vasculitis
    - Sickle Cell Anemia
  - INTRAVASCULAR HEMOLYSIS
    - C. Welchii Exotoxin
    - Complement—Autoimmune
    - G6PD and Drugs, Favism
    - Water, Heat

cell production as compared to the basal state. With hemolytic anemia, the production rate is usually 3 to 8 times normal, so that an index of 3 or more is taken as indicating excessive hemolysis. (It should be kept in mind that 3 to 5 days are required before the marrow can respond to anemia with a reticulocyte increase so that the rate of hemolysis is not accurately reflected by the reticulocyte index.) Corroborating evidence of hemolysis includes the findings of sphering and cell fragmentation in the blood smear, an increased bilirubin (predominantly indirect reacting) and an increased plasma lactic dehydrogenase (LDH).

A maturation abnormality (dyspoietic anemia) is characterized by evidence of increased cell death during development and/or by size changes of the circulating red cells. The reticulocyte index is less than 2 because most cells are destroyed before their emergence into circulation. The erythroid marrow is

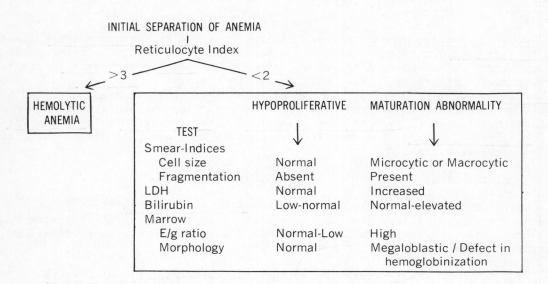

INITIAL SEPARATION OF ANEMIA
|
Reticulocyte Index

>3   <2

HEMOLYTIC ANEMIA		HYPOPROLIFERATIVE	MATURATION ABNORMALITY
TEST		↓	↓
Smear-Indices			
Cell size		Normal	Microcytic or Macrocytic
Fragmentation		Absent	Present
LDH		Normal	Increased
Bilirubin		Low-normal	Normal-elevated
Marrow			
E/g ratio		Normal-Low	High
Morphology		Normal	Megaloblastic / Defect in hemoglobinization

hyperplastic (E/G ratio 1:1 or greater), and there is an increase in indirect bilirubin and LDH. Red cell fragmentation on the blood smear (poikilocytosis), when associated with a reticulocyte index of less than 2, is strong evidence of ineffective erythropoiesis. This cell breakdown is presumed to occur as the abnormal cells attempt to enter the blood through the marrow sinusoidal wall. Size changes of the red cell are particularly helpful in indicating defective maturation: cell enlargement (exclusive of shift reticulocytes) is due to abnormalities in nuclear development, whereas decreased cell size (excluding fragmentation and sphering) is caused by abnormalities in hemoglobin synthesis. Cell size changes are proportionate to the degree of marrow stimulation by erythropoietin, and thus are more pronounced when anemia is severe. They may be identified by examining the blood smear or by determining the mean corpuscular volume (MCV). Each measurement has its own particular advantage (p. 55). A uniform change in size permits no comparison and thus may not be seen on the blood smear but is detected by cell indices. On the other hand, a small population of highly abnormal cells is more conspicuous under the microscope.

When cell size is increased, it is necessary to distinguish between the pathologic macrocytosis due to nuclear abnormalities and the physiologic macrocytosis associated with increased erythropoietin stimulation. The former cells are well filled with hemoglobin, have no hint of basophilia, and are frequently oval in shape. The latter, representing shift macrocytes, are slightly basophilic and slightly hypochromic. It has been suggested that a correction of about 2 μ^3 may be made for each per cent of reticulocytes present (3). However, the extent to which "shift" cells influence mean corpuscular volume depends not only on their number, but also on the extent of erythropoietin stimulation and iron supply (61). Another complication is the occasional occurrence of a dimorphic anemia, where combined defects in both nuclear and cytoplasmic development tend to cancel each other out in their effect on cell volume. In this circumstance, mean cell volume may be normal but hemoglobin concentration is decreased.

Hypoproliferative anemia is characterized by a low reticulocyte index (less than 2 times basal) without evidence of a maturation abnormality. Erythrocytes are usually of normal size, although there may be a moderate macrocytosis with a few shift cells if erythropoietin stimulation is increased. Bilirubin is frequently low (0.2 to 0.4 mg%). When the number of circulating granulocytes is normal, proliferation of the red cell precursors may be assessed from the aspirated marrow. With hypoproliferative anemia the E/G ratio is less than 1:1 and often less than 2:1. The detailed approach to this group of anemic patients will be considered first.

E. Differential Diagnosis of Hypoproliferative Anemia

Causes of hypoproliferation include an inadequate supply of iron for hemoglobin synthesis (often associated with blood loss), an intrinsic lesion of the marrow affecting erythroid stem cells, or a decrease in marrow stimulation by erythropoietin.

| Iron-Deficient Erythropoiesis |

Iron deficiency constitutes the most frequent cause of both hypoproliferative anemia and maturation abnormality. Since about half of iron-deficient erythropoiesis will be identified before any changes have occurred in red cell indices, many patients are initially considered to have a hypoproliferative disorder. The remaining patients will have a microcytic anemia and may be identified as having a maturation abnormality (see page 35). Precise methods are available for evaluating iron supply for erythropoiesis (62). The amount of iron available to the erythroid marrow is best expressed by the per cent saturation of transferrin (p. 63). Red cell protoporphyrin concentration reflects the adequacy of iron supply in relation to the needs of the erythroid marrow (43). While mean cell volume and erythrocyte hemoglobin

LABORATORY CRITERIA FOR THE DIAGNOSIS
OF IRON DEFICIENT ERYTHROPOIESIS

	Critical Level	Normal Range
Plasma Iron (μg/100 ml plasma)	<30	(50-180)
Transferrin Saturation (%)	<15	(20-60)
RBC Protoporphyrin (μg/100 ml RBC)	>100	(20-70)

concentration are very useful in detecting chronic iron deficiency, changes in cell indices do not occur for several months, and microcytic hypochromic anemia is not specific for iron deficiency.

Iron-deficient erythropoiesis is caused by either true iron deficiency or by inflammation, which blocks the internal recircuiting of iron. Iron deficiency may produce a spectrum of laboratory findings depending on the duration and severity (p. 16). With acute blood loss and large iron stores or supplemental iron administration, the reticulocyte index may be elevated to as much as 2 to 3 times normal, approaching the rate of erythropoiesis seen in hemolytic anemia. When bleeding has extended over a period of weeks, a hypoproliferative anemia with a reticulocyte index of about 1 is usually seen. In contrast to the normal

30

red cell indices of acute blood loss, long-standing iron deficiency anemia generates in addition a maturation defect with hypochromic, microcytic indices and some fragmentation (poikilocytosis).

IRON DEFICIENT ERYTHROPOIESIS

	SMEAR	SHIFT	RETIC INDEX	TRANSFERRIN (µg/100 ml)	SATURATION (%)	RE IRON STORES
RECENT BLEEDING	Normal	+ +	1-3	300-400	15-30	— to + +
IRON DEFICIENCY	Normal or microcytic/ hypochromic	+ +	1	350-500	5-12	—
INFLAMMATION	Normal	— to + +	1-2	150-300	10-20	+ + +

Once the presence of iron deficiency has been established, its cause must be sought (1-p.305). In the adult male this may be assumed to be bleeding, although infrequently gastrointestinal malabsorption, deposition of hemosiderin in the lungs or hemosiderinuria may produce deficiency. If external bleeding (epistaxis, bleeding hemorrhoids) is excluded by history, the source of bleeding is assumed to be the gastrointestinal tract. This assumption may be confirmed by guaiac tests on stool specimens in about half of the patients. However negative results by this test, even on several occasions, by no means exclude the possibility of GI blood loss, and a thorough study of the GI tract by x-ray and endoscopy is indicated. The possibility of malabsorption is best evaluated by an oral iron tolerance test, in which the increase in plasma iron level is determined after an oral dose of 100 mg of iron as ferrous sulfate. Hemosiderin sequestration in the lung and kidney may be demonstrated by microscopic examination of sputum or urinary sediment for iron.

CAUSES OF IRON DEFICIENCY

I Nutritional
   Female
   Infant
II Bleeding
   Menstrual
   Gastrointestinal
   Traumatic
   Other

III Malabsorption
   Post gastrectomy
   Sprue
IV Hemosiderin loss
   Pulmonary siderosis
   Hemosiderinuria

In the menstruating woman, pathologic causes of mild iron deficiency are difficult to distinguish from the nutritional iron deficiency found in 5-10% of females who are unable to maintain an adequate iron balance due to increased "normal" menstrual losses. The extent of menstrual bleeding cannot be accurately assessed by questioning but may be determined by direct measurement (63). Unfortunately, this procedure is usually not feasible, and the physician must make a decision based on the severity of the anemia, guaiac determinations, etc., whether the possibility of GI disease merits further investigation. In post-menopausal women, as in men, search for blood loss is always indicated. In infancy iron deficiency is commonly seen on a dietary basis and is usually accepted as such if the anemia is mild and if it occurs between the 4th and 24th months of life (earlier in the premature infant). Excepting nutritional iron deficiency, the cause of iron deficiency anemia is usually far more important than its treatment.

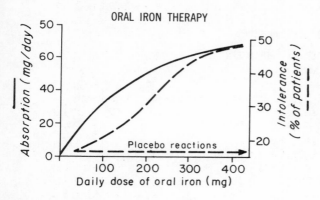

ORAL IRON THERAPY

Absorption (mg/day) — vertical axis: 50, 60, 40, 20, 0

Intolerance (% of patients) — right vertical axis: 50, 40, 30, 20

Placebo reactions

Daily dose of oral iron (mg) — horizontal axis: 100, 200, 300, 400

Iron deficiency is usually easily corrected through oral administration of iron. The dose is a compromise between giving sufficient iron to produce a prompt hematologic response but not enough to produce symptoms of iron intolerance (64). The usual dose of about 70 mg of ferrous iron given between meals in three doses (210 mg iron per day) should result in the daily absorption of 20-40 mg of iron and allow red cell production to reach 2 or 3 times normal.

Effectiveness of treatment is determined by the measure of blood hemoglobin concentration. An average increase of 0.2 g/day should occur after the third day, and an increase of over 2 gm% of circulating hemoglobin during a 3-week period is considered an adequate response. Measuring the reticulocyte response is usually of limited value except when the hemoglobin response is compromised by continued bleeding. Failure to respond may be due to unreliability of the patient in taking his medication, use of an unavailable (enteric coated) preparation, continued blood loss, the wrong diagnosis (inflammation, etc.) or malabsorption of iron. In event of malabsorption or rarely with intolerance to oral preparations, parenteral iron may be required. This form of treatment permits rapid reconstitution of iron stores, which would otherwise require 6-12 months of continued oral therapy. However, the use of parenteral iron is limited by rare febrile and anaphylactic reactions and the confusion created in subsequent evaluation of iron status.

The effects of inflammation on the erythron are very similar to those of true iron lack, since there is iron-deficient erythropoiesis in both conditions. However, some differences exist: the total iron binding capacity in iron deficiency is usually increased above normal, while it is decreased with inflammation. The per cent saturation of transferrin with inflammation is usually between 12 and 20, whereas, it is often below 10% with true iron deficiency. In inflammation the decrease in MCV and MCHC are usually no more than 10%, whereas they are often greater with chronic iron deficiency. Most decisive is the demonstration of hemosiderin particles in the reticuloenothelial cells of the marrow with inflammation in contrast to their absence with iron deficiency. More often than not, general clinical manifestations (fever, elevated sedimentation rate, etc.) indicate the presence of an inflammatory state. The anemia of inflammation is usually mild (hemoglobin over 10 gm%) and requires no treatment in itself. It will not respond to iron (p. 17). When more severe anemia is found with inflammation, other causes should be sought (hemolysis, maturation defect due to folate deficiency).

Failure of the erythron to proliferate occurs as part of a general disorder of the marrow (aplastic anemia) or

Marrow Failure

less commonly as an isolated finding (pure red cell aplasia) (1-p.207).
General marrow hypoplasia is probably best regarded as a stem cell disease
involving both uncommitted and committed stem cells. General categories of
causes are shown in the table below. Hypoplasia is suspected when levels of

CAUSES OF MARROW FAILURE

I Marrow Displacement	II Marrow Damage	III Intrinsic Lesion
Leukemia & lymphoma	Xray & toxic drugs	Congenital
Other neoplasm	Idiosyncratic reaction	Acquired
Myelofibrosis	Infection	Thymus related
Osteosclerosis		

circulating white cells and platelets as well as red cells are depressed. A
marrow aspiration or biopsy is generally carried out to differentiate aplastic
anemia from ineffective erythropoiesis and to detect morphologic abnormalities
within the marrow. Infiltration with neoplastic cells leads to therapeutic
considerations appropriate to the specific neoplastic process. The finding of
myelofibrosis requires further study to define the nature of the process and its
management, since it may be a manifestation of various myeloproliferative
processes and infiltrating malignancies, conditions with highly variable
prognoses. Localized osteosclerosis has similar implications.

The most important category is that in which marrow damage has been induced
by a toxic agent. A careful search is always made for an exposure to toxins.
While certain substances are well known to be myelotoxic (benzol, arsenic,
chemotherapeutic drugs employed in cancer therapy, etc.), their presence in
solvents, insecticides, and miscellaneous commercial chemicals may be difficult
to ascertain. The rare idiosyncratic reaction to a single drug is even more
difficult to recognize in a patient on multiple medications. However, such
drugs as chloromycetin, hydantoin derivatives, tolbutamide, and phenylbutasone,
are always suspect.

The severity of the aplastic process is best evaluated by the levels of
granulocytes and platelets in the circulating blood. The general treatment of
aplastic anemia involves first of all red cell transfusion to support the
circulating hemoglobin. Platelet transfusions may also be given when there is
thrombocytopenic bleeding. Unfortunately, isoantibodies develop which interfere
in time with further platelet support, and therefore platelet transfusion should
only be given for serious bleeding. Signs of infection should lead to a careful
search for pathogenic bacteria, and an early implementation of appropriate
antibiotic therapy. Some patients are helped by treatment with anabolic agents
in high dosage (2-3 mg/kg/day) (65). Response is slow, requiring at least 4
months of drug administration before a decision can be made about effectiveness.
Splenectomy is a further consideration in patients with an enlarged spleen.
While there is no general agreement about the indications for splenectomy, the
greater the size of the spleen the more likely that it has an adverse effect due
to sequestration and destruction of blood cells. In patients with life-
threatening aplasia of acute onset (granulocytes less than 100 and platelets
less than 5000/mm^3 of blood and an extremely hypocellular marrow), a search for
a histocompatible sibling should be carried out with the possibility of marrow
transplant in mind.

Pure red cell aplasia is usually considered due to unipotential (erythroid) stem cell damage, but may also be caused by a decreased erythropoietin production or interference with erythropoietin action. Drugs which produce aplastic anemia can also cause pure red cell aplasia. Red cell aplasia occurring at birth or in early infancy may respond to glucocorticoid administration. A few instances of antibody action against erythropoietin or against marrow elements have been described which respond to immunosuppressive drugs (66). Red cell aplasia may be found as a temporary phenomenon (aplastic crisis) in hemolytic states where temporary shutoff of red cell production produces a much greater fall in hemoglobin and is therefore detected.

| Erythropoietin Related Anemias |

Anemia due to decreased erythropoietin response has two general causes: 1) a disease impairing erythropoietin output from the kidney, and 2) an altered physiologic state where less hemoglobin is required for O_2 transport. The former category is the result of renal disease. Renal damage sufficient to produce anemia is associated with a BUN above 50 mg% and/or a creatinine elevation over 5 mg%. While moderate hemolysis may also be present, impaired production is the major defect. Both glomerular and tubular lesions interfere with erythropoietin production and result in a hypoproliferative anemia (67). The one exception is arteriolar damage which may lead to excretory renal failure and excessive red cell destruction without impairment of erythropoietin production or erythropoiesis (hemolytic-uremic syndrome). The hemoglobin in chronic renal disease usually does not go below about 6 gm%, and the anemia is well tolerated by the patient; only occasional patients require red cell transfusion. Androgens may improve erythropoietin output and on rare occasions may be indicated to obviate blood transfusion.

Physiologic alterations affecting O_2 transport usually result in only a moderate decrease in hemoglobin below the normal level. With single endocrine deficiencies (testosterone, glucocorticoids, or thyroxine) hemoglobin drops 1-4 gm%. Pituitary deficiency, with its effect on multiple target glands, may depress the hemoglobin by 3-6 gm%. The anemia is normochromic and normocytic without shift cells and with a normal red cell life span. Pregnancy probably falls in the same category, since hormonal factors are thought to cause a 1-2 gm decrease in hemoglobin concentration. With protein-calorie malnutrition, there is usually a 1-3 gm deficit in hemoglobin concentration and a somewhat greater decrease in red cell mass. Other causes, in particular iron and folate deficiency, should always be suspected when the hemoglobin is less than 11 gm%. With either endocrine disease or protein malnutrition, specific therapy is initially associated with a drop in hemoglobin concentration due to rapid expansion of plasma volume. After a lag of about one week there is reticulocytosis and an increase in hemoglobin concentration as the erythron expands.

A decrease in the affinity of hemoglobin for oxygen also causes decreased erythropoietin stimulation. The altered O_2 release has the effect of increasing the amount of O_2 carrying capacity required to deliver a normal amount of O_2 at a normal tissue O_2 tension. Such an effect is seen with certain amino acid substitutions in the globin chains of hemoglobin with or without an accompanying change in electrophoretic migration. Measurement of P_{50} is the only sure way to evaluate this possibility. Sometimes there is accompanying molecular instability which leads to increased red cell destruction. Indeed, in the group of hemolytic anemias with these combined abnormalities the concentration of hemoglobin is determined not by the amount of hemolysis but rather by the P_{50} (68). A decrease in hemoglobin affinity for oxygen may also result from a disorder of red cell metabolism such as pyruvate kinase deficiency which causes an increased concentration of red cell 2,3-DPG and thereby an increased availability of O_2 per gm hemoglobin.

F. Differential Diagnosis of Maturation Abnormalities

Maturation defects may be divided into cytoplasmic abnormalities, associated with a decrease in hemoglobin synthesis within the cell, and nuclear maturation abnormalities producing megaloblastic changes within the marrow and macrocytic changes in circulating red cells.

Iron deficiency differs from other types of microcytic anemia by having a low plasma iron, decreased saturation of transferrin, and a low ferritin level (p. 16&30). When there is a significant depression in mean corpuscular hemoglobin

> Impaired
> Hemoglobin
> Synthesis

concentration (less than 28%), its cause may be assumed to be iron deficiency. The only other conditions causing a similar decrease in MCHC are hemoglobin-opathies in which heme groups are progressively lost from the hemoglobin molecule and overhydration of the red cell occurs due to abnormalities of membrane pumps. However, these conditions are not associated with microcytosis. Iron-deficient erythropoiesis due either to true iron deficiency or infection is also distinguishable from other hemoglobin abnormalities by limited proliferation of erythroid cells and a low bilirubin.

The most common primary abnormality in globin synthesis is a quantitative impairment in either alpha or beta chain production as found in the thalassemias (1-p.328). The thalassemias differ in severity, depending in part on whether the patient is heterozygous or homozygous; however, there are other modifying factors so that the apparent genotype does not always coincide with the phenotype. In thalassemia minor (heterozygous) the only finding may be microcytosis and an increase in A_2 (α_2,δ_2) or fetal hemoglobin. In the more severe forms of thalassemia there is red cell fragmentation (poikilocytosis), stippling, and a hypochromic appearance in the blood smear. Medullary bone cavities are enlarged, causing facial deformities, and the spleen progressively enlarges through childhood due to its increased work in catabolizing red cells. Fetal hemoglobin (α_2,γ_2) is increased in the homozygous form of beta thalassemia, while hemoglobin H (β_4) is present in alpha thalassemia. Other thalassemia-like states (hemoglobin-E and hemoglobin Lepore) differ in that the hemoglobin molecules are structurally abnormal in addition to the decrease in chain

CRITERIA FOR DIAGNOSIS OF THALASSEMIA
1. Microcytic anemia without iron deficiency
2. Other family members involved
3. Ineffective erythropoiesis
4. Hemoglobin abnormalities

synthesis. With certain other abnormal hemoglobins, impaired heme attachment leads to intraerythrocytic hemoglobin destruction and consequent hypochromia, but little or no microcytosis. Since there is no known way of improving the synthesis of viable cells in these genetic abnormalities, therapy is supportive with red cell transfusions and appropriate treatment of complications such as pathologic fractures and hypersplenism.

Disorders of porphyrin synthesis are represented by the sideroblastic anemias (1-p.349). The abnormality is recognized by the presence of frequent mitochondrial sideroblasts in the marrow (p. 64). In some patients there is a general hypochromia and microcytosis on the blood smear; in others there is macrocytosis along with a minor population of hypochromic cells. The erythroid marrow is hyperplastic (E/G ratio > 1:1). Erythropoiesis is ineffective with little or no increase in circulating reticulocytes. The plasma iron is high and transferrin saturated. Protoporphyrin is usually low, although in a few patients an elevated protoporphyrin suggests an associated abnormality in heme chelatase activity. The heterogeneous group of conditions characterized by the finding of mitochondrial sideroblasts is best divided into 1) a hypochromic microcytic group having only an abnormality in hemoglobin (porphyrin) synthesis and 2) a normo- or macrocytic group with both nuclear and cytoplasmic abnormalities in red cell precursors. This is not an absolute distinction since some agents (alcohol) produce a selective abnormality in some patients and a combined lesion in others.

SIDEROBLASTIC ANEMIAS
I. Cytoplasmic Maturation Defect
   Hereditary (sex linked)
   Acquired:
      Idiopathic
      Secondary to alcohol, drugs or disease
II. Nuclear and Cytoplasmic Defect
   Alcoholism
   Other drugs and systemic diseases
   Intrinsic marrow disease

Isolated abnormalities in porphyrin synthesis occur in males as a hereditary (sex-linked) disorder, with parenchymal iron overload and the clinical manifestations of hemochromatosis. Some of these patients respond to pyridoxine and some do not, a difference which can only be determined by therapeutic trial. While sideroblastic changes have been reported in a great variety of diseases, including rheumatoid arthritis, carcinoma, myelofibrosis, hemolytic anemia, cutaneous porphyria, the reason for the abnormality in these conditions is unclear. A number of chemicals and drugs have been implicated, including alcohol, lead, isoniazid, and cycloserine, etc. Here the effect is presumed to be on porphyrin synthesis and more specifically, on ALA synthesis. Sideroblastic anemia of the pure cytoplasmic type also may develop in individuals of both sexes without known cause. Combined cytoplasmic-nuclear abnormalities are also found as a result of drugs and as an intrinsic marrow abnormality. There may be megaloblastic changes in the marrow, while the peripheral blood more often shows a macrocytic or dimorphic anemia than a microcytic anemia. Variable depressions in circulating levels of granulocytes and platelets are usually present. The most common condition is the combined abnormality found with alcoholism, where the megaloblastic change is associated with an abnormality in folate metabolism and there are variable degrees of sideroblastosis (69). Mitochondrial sideroblasts are also seen in refractory macrocytic (DiGuglielmo's) anemia. Many of these patients have alterations in platelet count (either increase of decrease) and moderate leukopenia.

Treatment of sideroblastic anemias involves first a consideration of removing the chemical agents or drugs which might be responsible. Lead poisoning may be suspected when heavy stippling is present in the blood film, and can be

investigated by determining blood and urine lead levels. If no specific
causative agent is found, empirical treatment is undertaken with pyridoxine (50
mg p.o. daily), since the most vulnerable step in porphyrin synthesis appears to
be the formation of ALA catalyzed by ALA synthetase, with pyridoxal phosphate as
a cofactor. Practical tests are not available by which responsiveness to
pyridoxine may be predicted in advance. Folic acid is usually tried empirically
particularly in patients with combined nuclear cytoplasmic abnormalities. The
majority of patients show no response to either of these agents.

The term "megaloblastosis" is considered synonymous

| Megaloblastic |
| Anemia |

with a nuclear maturation abnormality (1-p.249).
Megaloblastosis may be suspected from the presence of
true macrocytes and hypersegmented granulocytes in the blood smear or because of
macrocytic cell indices with an MCHC of 33 or above. The macrocytic cells of
megaloblastic anemia must be differentiated from shift macrocytes (p. 19) and
from the macrocytic anemia found with liver disease where red cells are of
uniform size and frequently targeted.

SPECTRUM OF MACROCYTIC INDICES

	NORMAL	STIMULATED ERYTHROPOIESIS	LIVER DISEASE	NUCLEAR DEFECT
MCV	90 ± 8	100 ± 10	105 ± 10	120 ± 30
MCHC	33 ± 2	31 ± 2	33 ± 2	33 ± 2
FRAGMENTATION	0	0	0	+
BILIRUBIN	Normal	Low-normal	Increased	Increased slightly

In megaloblastic anemia there is a marked variation in red cell size with
true macrocytes, often oval in shape, as well as many small cell fragments
(poikilocytes). The MCV is increased to as much as 150 μ^3. While the
reticulocyte index varies, it is usually extremely low (0.1 - 0.5). Bilirubin,
predominantly indirect, is increased (1-2 mg%), and LDH is often greater than
1000. Other findings in the peripheral blood smear include a reduction in white
cell and platelet counts, hypersegmented granulocytes, and platelets of variable
size. Marrow examination is usually revealing. The nuclear chromatin pattern
of both white and red cell precursors is finer
than usual, and the individual chromatin
particles more separated. The most
conspicuous finding in cells of the erythroid
series is the presence of a large immature-
appearing nucleus in association with a
hemoglobin-filled cytoplasm (nuclear-
cytoplasmic dissociation). In addition, in
the more mature nucleated red cells, nuclear
budding (Howell-Jolly bodies) is seen. These
various morphologic changes reflect the
essential nature of the disorder, an
abnormality of DNA metabolism which retards
nuclear development and mitosis without
affecting hemoglobin synthesis. Megaloblastic
changes are usually recognized in the blood

B_{12} DEFICIENCY
  Intrinsic factor deficiency
  Intestinal parasitism
  Malabsorption
  Dietary
  (Transport protein deficiency)
FOLATE DEFICIENCY
  Dietary
  Increased requirements
  Drug blockade (alcohol)
OTHER ABNORMALITIES IN DNA SYNTHESIS
  Extrinsic drugs
  Intrinsic mechanisms
  Congenital
  Acquired

smear and marrow smears with a hemoglobin concentration of less than 8 gm%. In milder anemia, megaloblastic changes may be undetectable or equivocal, the latter leading to the term "megaloblastoid." Over 90% of all cases of megaloblastic anemia are due to an abnormality of B_{12} or folate metabolism.

TESTS OF VITAMIN DEFICIENCY

VITAMIN B$_{12}$	NORMAL	POSSIBLE DEFICIENCY	DEFICIENCY
Plasma B$_{12}$ level (µµg/100 ml)	>200	100-200	<100
Urinary methylmalonate (mg/24 hrs.)	<4	4-10	>10
Gastric acidity after histamine (pH)	<3.5	—	>3.5
Schilling Test (8 hour plasma level- % dose/1% body wgt.)	>2	1-2	<1
FOLIC ACID			
Plasma Folate (mµg/ml)	>6	3-6	<3

Once a megaloblastic anemia is identified, tests are carried out to identify and distinguish between the treatable deficiencies of B_{12} and folate. The differentiation of these two deficiencies on clinical grounds is unreliable (70). Both substances produce similar abnormalities in the formed elements of blood. B_{12} deficiency alone produces neurologic damage, including posterior lateral cord degeneration, peripheral neuritis and central nervous system damage.

While a plasma level of more than 3 mµg/ml virtually excludes the possibility of folate deficiency, a low level by no means guarantees that diagnosis. Misleading values may be due to methodologic problems (antibiotics may affect microbiologic assays), and there are metabolic interrelations between folic acid and B_{12} which affect their plasma levels (71). Another useful test for B_{12} deficiency is the demonstration of dysfunction of biologically active B_{12} in tissues by measuring methylmalonate in the urine. The importance of making a specific diagnosis between the two deficiency states lies in the occurrence of disabling neurologic phenomenon in patients with B_{12} deficiency erroneously treated with folate, and because of different pathogenetic implications.

TREATMENT RESPONSE IN B$_{12}$ DEFICIENCY

In the patient who is not critically ill a therapeutic approach is often the most practical way to reach a specific diagnosis. Since there are nonspecific responses to larger doses of these vitamins, it is essential to limit the amount of folic acid given to 100 μg/day or the amount of vitamin B_{12} to 5 μg given intramuscularly daily. Folate therapy should be attempted first, since a normal diet may cause a folate response in the hospitalized individual with a nutritional deficiency. A response is documented by increases in reticulocyte count and hemoglobin concentration. In the more severely ill patient who may require immediate therapy with both drugs to insure a rapid recovery, blood should be drawn for serum levels of folate and B_{12} before treatment is instituted.

$\boxed{B_{12} \text{ Deficiency}}$ Impaired absorption is the usual cause of B_{12} deficiency. The absorptive process depends on: 1) elaboration by gastric parietal cells of intrinsic factor which binds B_{12} and protects it from enzymatic degradation in the gut; 2) the presence of receptors in the terminal ileum which take up B_{12} from intrinsic factor; and 3) absence of competitive consumption of B_{12} by bacteria or parasites in the small intestine. In the plasma, B_{12} is transported by transcobalamin-II. Another protein, transcobalamin-I, which binds much larger amounts, appears to derive its B_{12} from catabolism of white cells. Normally the body content of B_{12} is about 5000 μg, of which at least 2000 μg are in the liver. Since the daily turnover is 1-5 μg, it takes years for an individual starting with normal stores to become B_{12} deficient.

Once B_{12} deficiency occurs, the site and cause of malabsorption must be distinguished. The presence of free gastric acid after stimulation virtually excludes a gastric abnormality (except with a congenital defect manifested in childhood). The Schilling test, employing Co^{57}-labeled B_{12} is useful in determining the site of malabsorption. If B_{12} is absorbed only when intrinsic factor is added, deficient intrinsic factor may be assumed, focusing attention on the stomach. In elderly people the decreased synthesis of intrinsic factor due to gastric damage (atrophic gastritis, gastrectomy) is the most common cause of B_{12} deficiency. Autoantibodies may play an important role in causing intrinsic factor deficiency in younger patients. If absorption is shown to be inadequate when intrinsic factor is added to the Co^{57} B_{12} test dose, an abnormality of the small bowel is probable and appropriate x-ray studies should be carried out. Malabsorption may result from disease of the ileum (regional enteritis, sprue) or may be produced by overgrowth of bacterial organisms in the small bowel (blind loop or diverticuli) with B_{12} consumption by these organisms. Other causes of ileal malfunction include long-standing myxedema, and the effects of certain drugs (colchicine, paraminosalicylic acid, etc.). In a few instances the malabsorptive process may be effectively treated. A gluten-free diet relieves the symptoms of gluten enteropathy, and antibiotics may reduce small bowel sepsis. However, in most instances B_{12} malabsorption is uncorrectable, and replacement therapy is required. After a preliminary series of parenterally administered loading doses, 100 μg IM of B_{12} every 3-4 weeks is adequate maintenance.

$\boxed{\text{Folate Deficiency}}$ Dietary folate derived from green, leafy vegetables occurs as polyglutamate compounds which are broken down by conjugases within the intestine. The efficiency of this process and thus the amount of available folate from diet is not known. At least 50 µg of absorbed folate is required each day to prevent tissue deficiency. Body stores amount to about 5000 µg, so that it takes 3 or 4 months to develop a deficiency state after intake is interrupted. The primary metabolic function of folate is in one carbon transfer reactions, in which the reduced form (N^5-methyl tetrahydrofolate) functions as a coenzyme. The inability to synthesize thymidine as a result of folate deficiency interferes with the formation of DNA and results in a megaloblastic anemia.

Folic acid deficiency occurs with inadequate dietary intake, impaired absorption and increased body requirements for folate. A several-fold increase in folate requirements with pregnancy, infection, general neoplastic disease and hemolytic anemia leads to an increased incidence of megaloblastic anemia in these conditions. Patients with increased folate requirements should probably be on continuous folate therapy (1 mg/day). The most common drug with an adverse effect on folate metabolism is alcohol, reducing folate intake by substituting for other food and impairing internal folate transport. A number of other drugs with apparently adverse effects include in particular anticonvulsant drugs (diphenylhydantoin, phenobarbital and primadone), glutethimide, isoniazid and cycloserine, and mestranol. When there are toxic effects from these drugs, oral folate re-establishes an adequate folate supply. However, this reversal does not occur when folate antagonists are used in cancer therapy (methotrexate) or with pyrimethamine given as an antimalarial drug. Their toxic effects can be reversed by treatment with folinic rather than folic acid.

Megaloblastic anemia may be caused by abnormalities other than folate and B_{12} deficiency. Extrinsic agents, in particular chemicals used in cancer therapy affect nucleic acid metabolism, producing megaloblastic changes. Included are 6-mercaptopurine, hydroxyurea, daunomycin, ara-C, 5-fluoro-uracil, 6-azauridine, etc. There are also hereditary abnormalities affecting nucleic acid metabolism, including orotic aciduria and formininotransferase deficiency, whose recognition leads to effective treatment. Finally, there is a rather large group of patients with acquired intrinsic abnormalities of the marrow which cause a somewhat similar morphologic picture, presumably also due to a defect of nuclear maturation. The name DiGuglielmo's anemia (refractory anemia) is given to this group of conditions; it implies little more than a mcacrocytic anemia in which the erythroid marrow is hyperplastic with megaloblastic and occasionally sideroblastic changes. In a number of patients with DiGuglielmo's anemia, the marrow morphology changes to the blastic picture of acute leukemia, so that the presence of an increased number of blasts is significant. While the condition is generally unresponsive to therapy, some patients respond partially to folate or pyridoxine, and these agents are therefore given a trial. Prognosis is usually best defined by the stability or progressive decline in granulocyte and platelet levels.

G. The Differential Diagnosis of Hemolytic Anemia

Red cell destruction may occur from a great variety of causes. In a significant number of patients the etiology remains obscure (72). Information concerning drug intake or toxin exposure, associated disease, familial involvement, splenic size and laboratory findings all provide entry points for the specialist to reach a diagnosis. The physician approaches hemolytic anemia mindful of the importance of recognizing the mechanism of destruction (immune,

40

HEMOLYTIC DISEASE

I Intravascular hemolysis
   Mechanical
   Osmotic
   Chemicals
   Complement damage
II Fragmentation hemolysis
   Sickle cell anemia
   Arteriolar damage
   Consumption coagulopathy
   Heart valve prosthesis

III RE Destruction
   Immune hemolysis
   Heinz body anemias-
    metabolic
    hemoglobinopathy
   Red cell membrane abnormalities-
    hereditary spherocytosis
   Anaerobic glycolytic abnormalities-
    pyruvate kinase deficiency, etc.

splenic, oxidative) because of its therapeutic implications and the importance of identifying causative drugs and toxins so that further exposure can be prevented (73). This manual will examine hemolytic disorders according to the destruction pattern, since the possibilities are thereby reduced to a more manageable number. The three categories of red cell damage in decreasing order of severity include: 1) intravascular hemolysis, characterized by a plasma hemoglobin level of over 30 mg% and hemoglobinuria, 2) red cell fragmentation identified by the presence of red cell fragments on smear and hemosiderinuria, and 3) extravascular hemolysis which shows very little beyond an increased reticulocyte index reflecting the increased red cell turnover.

Intravascular hemolysis is recognized by the presence of visible amounts of free hemoglobin in plasma and/or urine. Care must be taken to differentiate hemoglobinuria from other

> Intravascular
> Hemolysis

causes of urine coloration (myoglobin, porphobilinogen, dipyrolles, and urobilinogen) and particularly from hematuria. True hemoglobinuria is accompanied by visible hemoglobinemia. Severe damage to a certain number of red cells is implicit with the demonstration of intravascular hemolysis, but the number of destroyed red cells is not necessarily large. The trauma of walking on a hard pavement (march hemoglobinuria) or the introduction into circulation of distilled water used as an irrigating fluid during transurethral prostatectomy may produce hemoglobinuria but little anemia. Complement damage with extensive intravascular as well as extravascular red cell destruction is caused by intrinsic red cell lesions (paroxysmal nocturnal hemoglobinuria), and by antibodies (cold and warm auto- and alloantibodies) which attach complement to the red cell membrane. Chemicals such as arsine damage red cells by reacting with sulfhydryl groups; the alpha toxin of C. welchii contains a lecithinase which acts on lipoprotein complexes of the red cell membrane; and fava beans or oxidative drugs damage cells when there is defective red cell aerobic metabolism (G6PD) deficiency). Sudden severe intravascular hemolysis without apparent cause is particularly suggestive of an autoimmune, complement-dependent hemolysis or, in the female, of abortion infected with C. welchii. Paroxysmal nocturnal hemoglobinuria is more likely with chronic hemoglobinuria. It is identified by the sucrose or acid hemolysis tests.

The fragmentation syndrome represents a lesser degree of intravascular breakdown. There is a mechanical destruction of circulating red cells with liberation of sufficient

> Fragmentation
> Hemolysis

hemoglobin to deplete haptoglobin and hemopexin, resulting in methemalbuminemia and hemosiderinuria. However, free hemoglobin in the plasma does not usually

41

rise above 30 mg% and there is no overt hemoglobinuria. For diagnosis, the
presence of fragmented red cells on the blood smear (p. 57) is less reliable
than the demonstration of hemosiderin in desquamated tubular cells of a
concentrated urine specimen. Fragmentation may be caused by increased cell
rigidity imposed by sickle hemoglobin, or as the result of Heinz body
phagocytosis. Most often, fragmentation hemolysis is due to abnormal vascular
surfaces, particularly arteritis as in malignant hypertension, immune
disease, or certain infections. The hemolytic uremic syndrome is the result of
damage to arterioles of the kidney. Consumptive coagulopathy, with fibrin
deposits on vessel walls secondary to arterial damage or intravascular clotting,
may produce red cell fragmentation (74). Valve prostheses are also capable of
breaking cells. An interesting complication of both fragmentation and
intravascular hemolysis when of long duration is the development of iron
deficiency due to loss of large amounts of iron as hemosiderin in the urine (up
to 20 mg/day).

| RE Hemolysis | Destruction of red cells by the RE system predominates in virtually all hemolytic anemias, even those classifed as intravascular hemolysis or fragmentation. However, in those anemias ascribed to RE breakdown, there is relatively little destruction in the vascular compartment. Haptoglobin is frequently depleted, but free hemoglobin levels are only slightly increased and there is no significant methemalbuminemia or hemosiderinuria. This group of conditions characterized by reticuloendothelial destruction is by far the largest category of hemolytic anemia and often causes considerable difficulty in reaching a specific diagnosis.

In working up an anemia of this type, it is especially important to search
for some genetic abnormality, external agent, or disease capable of producing
red cell destruction. Racial derivation and family history of anemia may suggest
a genetic disorder. Certain chemicals act as harmful oxidants in individuals
with impaired aerobic glycolysis (G6PD deficiency); other chemicals act through
an immune mechanism, while still others have direct destructive effect on red
cells. Enlargement of lymph nodes suggests disease of the immune system whereas
an enlarged spleen is merely consistent with increased red cell destruction in
that organ. Diseases such as lupus erythrematosus and lymphatic leukemia, as
well as certain infections (mycoplasma, infectious mononucleosis, cytomegalic
disease) are frequently associated with autoimmune hemolytic anemia. In the
absence of specific clues, an attempt is made by laboratory procedures to
identify the disorder in one of three main categories.

| Autoimmune Hemolytic Anemia | Autoimmune disorders are identified by a positive Coombs (antiglobulin) test indicating the adherence of immunoglobulin or complement to the red cell surface (75). A coating of IgG alone can lead to phagocytosis by RE cells which recognize specific sites on the Fc fragment of the IgG heavy chain. IgG and IgM may also fix complement to the red cell membrane. When this occurs, the Coombs test is positive only when the antiglobulin serum contains antibodies against C3 and/or C4. Some patients with immune hemolytic anemia do not have a positive Coombs test because the amount of antibody attached to red cell surfaces is too small to be detected (less than 500 antibody molecules per cell). The immune nature of the process may then be inferred only from a response to glucocorticoids.

Autoantibodies appear in response to infections and drugs as well as in association with benign and malignant disorders of the immune system. Drugs produce an autoantibody reaction in several ways: the drug and its antibody may form a complex which is loosely attached to the red cell, the drug may function as a haptene, or the drug may stimulate production of an antibody which reacts with red cell antigens. General immune disorders such as lupus, rheumatoid arthritis, sarcoid, periarteritis, regional enteritis, etc. are associated with the production of autoantibodies against red cells as well as other tissues. Patients with malignancies of the immune system, especially lymphocytic leukemia, commonly have demonstrable red cell autoantibodies or a hemolytic anemia responsive to glucocorticoids. Some clue to the underlying disease is provided by the specificity of the antibody. For example, IgM (cold agglutinins) usually have I or i specificity and are often caused by mycoplasma infections of lymphoproliferative disorders. About 1/3 of patients with infectious mononucleosis develop anti-i antibodies. IgG antibodies against an antigen in the P system are found in the Donath-Landsteiner cold hemolysis syndrome.

Long-standing autoimmune hemolytic anemia poses an appreciable threat to life. In general, one may expect 1/3 of the patients to die within 2 years, 1/3 to have continuing disease, and 1/3 to be cured by treatment. Death is most commonly related to intractable anemia, infection, or pulmonary embolism and other cardiovascular complications. Steroids produce initial remissions in about 85% of cases, but when the drug is stopped, the remission continues in only a small proportion. As a rule, steroids are more effective against IgG antibodies than against IgM antibodies, although this is not invariably true. Splenectomy is successful in curing about 1/3 of patients; the potential effect of this procedure may be evaluated to some extent by monitoring the radioactivity of Cr^{51} tagged cells in vivo. Accumulation of activity in the spleen is evidence for, and lack of accumulation against, a therapeutic result. Cytotoxic drugs (Imuran, chlorambucil, Cytoxan) are sometimes helpful in arresting the hemolytic process in patients with chronic lymphocytic leukemia and in patients with no known underlying disease who have been splenectomized and in whom the maintenance dose of prednisone required to control the hemolytic process is so large as to be toxic.

Oxidative destruction of hemoglobin (1-p.391) occurs in a group of disorders in which hemoglobin is abnormally vulnerable to denaturation, either because oxidative glycolysis is

Heinz Body Anemias

impaired or because the hemoglobin molecule is structurally unstable. With severe impairment of the hexosemonophosphate shunt pathway there is chronic hemolytic anemia; more often, exposure to some oxidant drug or infection is needed to produce a time-limited hemolytic episode. The hallmark of oxidative damage is the presence of Heinz bodies in wet preparations of red cells treated with brilliant cresyl violet. Since aggregates of denatured hemoglobin are rapidly removed from the red cell in vivo by the RE cells of the spleen, the diagnosis may be missed if studies are not carried out while the hemolytic process is still present. When hemolysis occurs in association with drug intake or infection, a latent deficiency in oxidative metabolism due to reduced activity of glucose 6-phosphate dehydrogenase (G6PD) is likely. The structural locus for G6PD is on the X chromosome, so deficiency occurs more often in males than in females. Specific tests for G6PD activity are available, but may give normal results if the G6PD deficient cells (i.e., the older cells) are already destroyed. The abnormality can only be diagnosed later, when the young red cells have grown older or by studies in other family members. A variety of different G6PD abnormalities exists, some of which, i.e. the Mediterranean variety, are capable of producing very severe hemolytic episodes, while other, i.e. the Negro variety, are associated with mild hemolytic reactions on exposure to oxidant agents. Therapy consists of removing those agents (including infection) and providing red cell support during severe hemolytic reactions. An <u>unstable hemoglobin</u> may cause either chronic or episodic hemolysis. The denatured hemoglobin in circulating red cells may not be evident because of splenic removal, but a heat stability or alcohol precipitation test will demonstrate the molecular abnormality.

| Congenital Defects of Membrane and Metabolism | Congenital disorders of the red cell membrane and of metabolic systems constitute a third category of extravascular hemolytic anemias. Generally, these conditions are considered after excluding intravascular hemolysis, aerobic metabolic disorders (Heinz body anemias), and autoimmune abnormalities |

(Coombs positive hemolytic anemias). Family history of a hemolytic disorder suggests an intrinsic red cell lesion of membrane or anaerobic metabolism. An initial distinction between spherocytic and non-spherocytic anemias is made on the basis of a blood smear, and, if necessary, an osmotic fragility test. <u>Hereditary spherocytosis</u> is one of the most rewarding conditions to recognize because splenectomy is nearly always effective treatment. This condition, thought to represent an inherited abnormality of membrane protein, produces a variable degree of sphering, sometimes difficult to detect. The MCHC is usually increased, reflecting membrane loss. The osmotic fragility and autohemolysis tests are helpful (p. 73). Hereditary elliptocytosis may or may not be associated with a hemolytic process but is easily identified on the blood smear. Other abnormalities associated with membrane regulation of intracellular electrolytes can cause increased fragility through overhydration of the cell (76).

Abnormalities of the Embden-Meyerhof pathway do not cause sphering but the cells show irregular surfaces. The autohemolysis test may show very mild to greatly increased hemolysis. Pyruvate kinase deficiency is the most frequent abnormality of this group, followed by glucose phosphate isomerase deficiency. While screening tests are available to detect enzyme inactivity, results are often equivocal. If the possibility of an enzyme defect cannot be ruled out, it may be useful to measure the O_2 dissociation curve and/or red cell DPG level. Enzyme defects which act before production of 2,3-DPG decrease its level, causing a left shift in the O_2 dissociation curve (hexokinase, GPI, PFK, etc.) With lesions below this metabolic step (including PK deficiency) the DPG level is high, and the O_2 curve is shifted to the right. Intrinsic red cell lesions must be distinguished from hemolytic disorders associated with irregular cell surfaces due to an extrinsic defect, as may be found with liver disease, renal disease, or abetalipoproteinemia.

| General Therapy | In management of hemolytic anemias, identifying the specific etiologic agent may lead to a cure by removal of the offending drug or by specific treatment as in the case of some infections. |

Autoimmune processes may be more generally approached by the use of glucocorticoids and immunosuppressive agents or by splenectomy. The need for <u>transfusion</u>

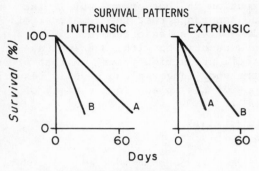

SURVIVAL PATTERNS

INTRINSIC   EXTRINSIC

A = Normal cells in patient
B = Patient cells in normal

support is to be considered in patients with evidence of inadequate O_2 supply (p. 23) or to prevent development of hypoxia in patients with severe acute hemolysis. The RE system has the capacity to catabolize as much as 20% the normal circulating red cell mass per day, and if all red cells have prominent Heinz bodies, this rate of destruction can be anticipated. The effectiveness of transfusion depends on whether the hemolytic mechanism is intrinsic or extrinsic to the red cell. Cr^{51} tagging of transfused cells provides evidence to answer this question. On some occasions when an extrinsic process is operating (cold autoimmune hemolytic anemia) the patient's own population of red cells may be more resistant to hemolysis than those transfused, in which case transfusion is associated with a rise in red cell destruction. In an intrinsic hemolytic process when the patient becomes acutely anemic due to decreased marrow function (aplastic crisis), the knowledge that transfused cells will live a normal life span is helpful.

The role of the spleen is important to evaluate in any chronic hemolytic anemia for two reasons: 1) in certain hemolytic anemias (hereditary spherocytosis) excessive red cell destruction is virtually limited to the spleen, and removal of this organ stops significant hemolysis; 2) increased red cell destruction by the spleen leads to progressive splenomegaly which may eventually cause increased destruction of normal cells as well as abnormal. The extent of

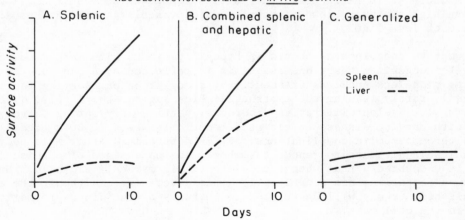

RBC DESTRUCTION LOCALIZED BY IN VIVO COUNTING

A. Splenic   B. Combined splenic and hepatic   C. Generalized

Spleen ———
Liver — — —

red cell destruction within the spleen is best determined by tagging the patient's cells with Cr^{51} and determining the in vivo uptake over the spleen, liver and heart. Absence of selective splenic uptake makes it unlikely that the

45

hemolytic process will be alleviated by splenectomy. Increased localization in the spleen indicates increased red cell destruction in that organ, but in the case of autoimmune hemolytic anemias, given no assurance that the remainder of the RE system may not take over the destruction after splenic removal. The presence of an enlarged red cell pulp is always associated with some increase in red cell destruction and, even when some red cell production occurs in that organ (myelofibrosis with metaplasia), removal of the very large spleen usually results in a more favorable red cell balance. The role of the spleen in a variety of hemolytic states is shown below.

SPLENIC DESTRUCTION IN HEMOLYTIC ANEMIAS
BY SURVIVAL MEASUREMENTS

MARKED	MODERATE	UNIMPORTANT
Hereditary spherocytosis	Hypersplenism	Intravascular hemolytic syndromes
Ovalocytosis	Certain unstable hemoglobins	
Autoimmune disease (IgG)	**Autoimmune disease**	Fragmentation disorders
	Certain abnormalities in anaerobic glycolysis	Defects in aerobic glycolysis
		Autoimmune disease (IgM)

II. POLYCYTHEMIA

A. Clinical Manifestations

The clinical manifestations of polycythemia are so variable and inconsistent that they have little diagnostic value. An extremely high hematocrit (over 70%) is associated with general malaise, fatigue, and headache, presumably because the high viscosity impairs blood flow and thereby O_2 supply. Increased blood viscosity requires increased cardiac work and may precipitate insufficiency in the individual with borderline cardiac function. Arterial hypertension with generalized arteriosclerosis is frequently observed in polycythemia vera. However, if polycythemia is compensatory to hypoxia, as with high altitude, there is a decrease in peripheral arterial resistance which results in low rather than high systemic blood pressure. Cardiovascular complications are therefore much less likely.

Consumptive coagulopathy occurs in hypoxic patients with marked polycythemia secondary to congenital heart disease; this is reflected by a decrease in circulating platelets and less frequently by a depletion of clotting factors (fibrinogen), rarely leading to hemorrhage. Bleeding due to platelet dysfunction also occurs with myeloproliferative disorders, particularly during surgery. In patients with cardiac disease an elevated hemoglobin seems to be a predisposing factor to thromboembolic complications. It is debatable whether mild polycythemia in itself disposes to venous thrombosis in the absence of cardiac failure, but this is undoubtedly true when the hematocrit is markedly elevated. Special vascular manifestations are seen in polycythemia vera (77); although the cause is not established, it may well be related to features of the disease other than the increase in red cell mass.

B. Detection of Polycythemia

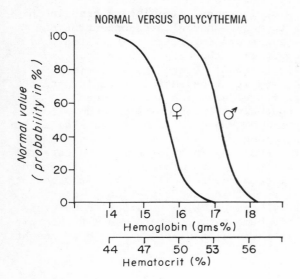

NORMAL VERSUS POLYCYTHEMIA

The laboratory diagnosis of polycythemia is based on the hemoglobin concentration. An arbitrary upper limit is 17.5 gm for males and 16 gm for females at sea level, but the actual designation of polycythemia is contingent on matters previously discussed in relation to anemia (p. 24). The decision must be made with each patient as to whether the likelihood of a polycythemic state is sufficiently great and its cause sufficiently obscure to require investigation. The probability of polycythemia as shown in the accompanying figure is based on an overall frequency of 4% in both men and women. The physiologic norm for the individual is increased by altitude or by any condition in which the arterial O_2 saturation is decreased. In other words, the need for hemoglobin rises as available O_2 content of the blood decreases, regardless of the cause.

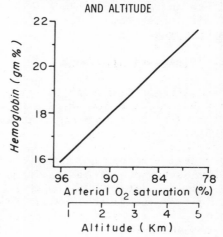

HEMOGLOBIN RELATIONSHIP TO HYPOXIA AND ALTITUDE

C. General Therapeutic Considerations

The immediate therapeutic implications of a high hemoglobin concentration are few until the cell/plasma imbalance becomes extreme. Treatment depends primarily upon whether the polycythemia is due to a decrease in plasma volume (relative polycythemia) or to a true increase in red cell mass. The former may be rapid in onset and symptoms then usually relate to the decrease in total blood volume. Management is directed at expanding the plasma volume by the most specific means possible (saline for salt depletion, plasma when there has been a plasma loss or steroids for abnormal vascular permeability).

The increased red cell mass of true polycythemia requires time to develop (unless produced by excess red cell transfusion). Treatment is urgent only when the degree of polycythemia is marked (hematocrit greater than 70 or hemoglobin greater than 23 gm%), or when there are cardiovascular complications. It is desirable to establish whether hypoxia is present, and if so, its severity. When

there is an increase in red cell mass and total blood volume unaccompanied by
arterial desaturation, the volume-viscosity overload can be reduced by
phlebotomy. Patients with hypoxia require an increased circulating hemoglobin
concentration, and care must be taken not to reduce hemoglobin concentration
below the optimal level. Volume considerations are important in both the
initial appraisal of the patient and in evaluating the effects of phlebotomy.
Especially in the aged patient with arteriosclerosis, there are as serious
hazards of hypovolemia as of polycythemia, and it is essential to manipulate the
blood volume within safe limits. Consider the elderly man who has been
exercising excessively on a hot day, who suddenly becomes comatose and is found
to have an increased hematocrit. He may well have pre-existing polycythemia, but
the cutaneous and muscular vasodilatation, along with excessive sweating, may
have rendered his blood volume inadequate, resulting in hypotension and cerebral
thrombosis. In the management of such a patient, it is often more important to
maintain an adequate blood volume than to reduce the red cell mass, although both
are important considerations. Intravascular clotting and depletion of clotting
factors leading to bleeding may occasionally occur at high hematocrits but rarely
constitute an emergency; platelet levels and hemostatic factors usually return to
normal with phlebotomy. Other causes of intravascular clotting should be sought
if the bleeding disorder is severe.

D. Diagnostic Approach

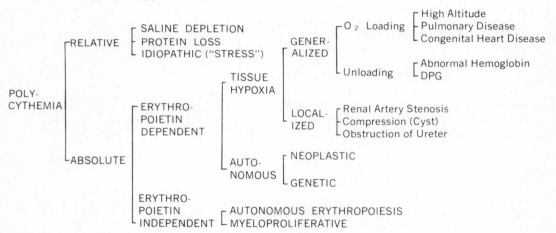

The working classification of polycythemia is shown in the figure above.
While this approach may be employed in obscure instances of chronic polycythemia,
there are often clues which permit the physician to bypass the initial blood
volume determination required in this branching format. Thus, hypoxia is the
most common cause of polycythemia, and frequently cyanosis or symptoms of
pulmonary disease suggest the need of determining the arterial O_2 saturation.
Likewise, the presence of a palpable spleen accompanied by increases in
circulating platelets and/or white cells suggest the diagnosis of polycythemia
vera. In this manual, however, a general approach will be undertaken on the
assumption that such specific clues may not exist.

Once the individual has been selected for study because of a high hemoglobin, it is important to consider the <u>plasma volume</u>. The most common cause of temporary polycythemia is fluid loss secondary to the use of diuretics. Nausea, vomiting, diarrhea and excessive sweating represent other more evident causes of fluid loss. High capillary pressure (increased catecholamines or heart failure) or increased vascular permeability (burns, anaphylaxis) may temporarily decrease plasma volume and increase hemoglobin concentration. The clinical setting permits an understanding of the cause of the problem in such situations and dictates a logical therapeutic approach as previously discussed (p. 48).

> Relative
> Polycythemia

Plasma volume depletion in conjunction with a normal red cell mass is also seen as a chronic state (78). The physiology of this condition, referred to as "stress polycythemia" because of its frequent occurrence in patients with ulcer and cardiovascular disease, is poorly understood. The same blood volume change is seen with Cushing's disease. The recognition of a decreased plasma volume as a cause of increased hemoglobin concentration is important in respect to diagnosis and treatment. Such patients react unfavorably to phlebotomy and are believed to be at risk for developing cardiovascular complications.

True polycythemia is defined as an increase in both hemoglobin concentration and red cell mass. Excluding red cell transfusion as a cause, true polycythemia is the result of hypoxia or some abnormality in regulation of erythropoiesis. The normal behavior of erythropoietin has been described elsewhere (p. 18). Any decrease in O_2 in blood going to the kidney generates an increased erythropoietin level in plasma, resulting in increased erythropoiesis and a rise in hemoglobin concentration. Increased hemoglobin affinity for oxygen also increases the erythropoietin output and leads to increased hemoglobin concentration. On the other hand, changes in blood flow over a wide range cause little change in erythropoietin output, presumably because renal blood supply and renal oxygen requirements change in parallel. Thus, in the cardiac patient, sodium regulation is impaired before erythropoietin is affected, and any marked increase in hemoglobin concentration suggests either disequilibrium of the plasma and red cell mass due to diuresis or some associated problem causing a decrease in arterial O_2 saturation (cor pulmonale with secondary heart failure).

> True
> Polycythemia

Insight into abnormalities in response of the erythron is gained by measuring erythropoietin output at different hemoglobin concentrations in various types of polycythemia (45). In the usual patient with hypoxic polycythemia, the erythropoietin response curve is displaced to the right. With autonomous erythropoiesis (polycythemia vera), erythropoietin output is suppressed and with autonomous

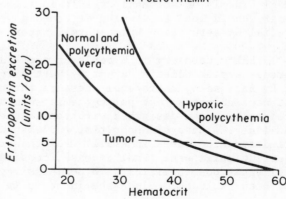

ERYTHROPOIETIN RESPONSE TO PHLEBOTOMY IN POLYCYTHEMIA

production of erythropoietin (hormone-producing tumor), the erythropoietin level appears independent of the hemoglobin concentration. It would be of great assistance in the diagnostic approach to polycythemia if erythropoietin concentration and its change with phlebotomy could be measured, but at the present time this is not practical as a routine procedure.

| Hypoxic Polycythemia | The physician must first separate appropriate increases in hemoglobin concentration from those that are unphysiologic (79). An appropriate increase has to be the result of some

decrease in the O_2 supply. A decrease in <u>arterial O_2 saturation</u>, when present, provides the most clearcut supporting evidence, but the degree of hypoxia demonstrated by a single arterial sample may correlate poorly with the degree of polycythemia. Ventilatory activity may be stimulated during the time of blood sampling, concealing an otherwise depressed O_2 saturation. Activity and sleep may produce a degree of arterial desaturation not otherwise observed. A decreased arterial O_2 tension can be excluded as the cause of polycythemia only after these possibilities have been evaluated. The poor correlation between arterial desaturation and polycythemia is particularly evident in chronic pulmonary disease. In such patients a number of factors can affect O_2 exchange: the 24-hour O_2 saturation, modification in acid-base balance which alters the affinity of hemoglobin for O_2, complicating infections and iron deficiency. If a decrease in arterial O_2 saturation is demonstrated, a detailed study of pulmonary function or a search for pulmonary or cardiac shunts is indicated. The only management consideration with such hypoxic polycythemias is whether the hemoglobin concentration is optimal for the decreased amount of available O_2. There is no practical way to make this determination other than by evaluating the symptomatic status of the patient after a trial of phlebotomy. It is well to determine from the plasma iron and transferrin saturation whether iron deficiency has limited the erythropoietic response.

Certain rare genetic disorders of the red cell affect O_2 release. Hemoglobinopathies in which the abnormal hemoglobin has a left-shifted dissociation curve have the same effect as metabolic abnormalities of the red cell in which the DPG level is low. These possibilities may be suspected by a familial incidence of polycythemia and verified by P_{50} determination. In such situations the altered hemoglobin concentration compensates for the decreased O_2 availability and no treatment is required. Methemoglobinemia and carboxy-hemoglobinemia occasionally result in raised hemoglobin levels. Cyanosis in the former should lead to studies of blood gases, which will show a decreased arterial O_2 saturation but a normal arterial O_2 pressure.

A third category is hypoxia of one kidney. Experimentally it is possible to increase erythropoietin output by partially obstructing renal arterial blood flow and by increasing intrarenal pressure through ureteral ligation. Clinical evidence indicates that polycythemia secondary to unilateral renal disease is rare; it has been described with renal artery obstruction, with cystic disease of the kidney, with pyelonephritis, and with ureteral obstruction, but the number of well-documented cases is small. For this reason and because of the difficulty in detecting unilateral renal disease, consideration of this cause is usually left until other possibilities of hypoxic polycythemia and autonomous erythropoiesis have been excluded. Since the increase in red cell mass is inappropriate in this condition, treatment of the polycythemia consists of reducing the red cell mass and hemoglobin concentration to normal by phlebotomy.

Polycythemia may also result from the autonomous output of erythropoietin. When there is no evidence of hypoxia or autonomous erythropoiesis, a careful search should be made for an erythropoietin-producing neoplasm. Hypernephroma, angioblastoma of the cerebellum, and hepatoma are the most frequent tumors responsible, although others have been described (80). An unusual condition of autonomous erythropoietin production occurs as a familial disorder without demonstrable anatomic lesions (81).

> Autonomous
> Erythropoietin
> Production

Polycythemia may also be caused by proliferative disease of the marrow (1-p.527). Polycythemia vera is usually characterized by an increase in all marrow elements and by splenomegaly; indeed, the diagnosis of polycythemia vera should probably not be made if the erythron alone is involved. In this condition red cell production is independent of the action of erythropoietin and no erythropoietin is present in blood or urine. The O_2 dissociation curve is normal or slightly displaced to the left and 2,3-DPG is not increased (in contrast to the increase found in hypoxic polycythemia). Additional clinical features useful in reaching the diagnosis include the presence of pruritus, particularly after a hot bath, acrocyanosis, peripheral vascular disease, an elevated uric acid and occasionally manifestations of gout. Laboratory abnormalities include increased granulocytes and more important, an increase in circulating basophils to 200 or more (normal $40/mm^3$), elevated leukocyte alkaline phosphatase, an increase in blood platelets with variation in platelet size, and other evidence of marrow stromal disease. When red cell increase constitutes the major problem, phlebotomy is effective treatment. The objective of phlebotomy is not only to normalize the red cell mass but also to impose iron deficiency. After this has been done, one phlebotomy every three months is usually sufficient to maintain a normal hemoglobin. When platelets and/or white cells are affected, chemotherapy may be employed with such myelosuppressive agents as myleran or chlorambucil.

> Autonomous
> Erythropoiesis

Although mechanisms for production of polycythemia are well understood, it should not be inferred that the differential diagnosis of polycythemia is easy. As suggested by the previous discussion, careful evaluation of blood volume, arterial O_2 saturation, P_{50}, and of kidney structure and function by excretory urography and possibly renal angiograms may be needed. The separation of relative and true polycythemia by blood volume determinations seems simple but in fact the results are not always definite and at times are misleading. Hypoxic polycythemia due to a decreased O_2 saturation is not always apparent from determinations made in the basal awake state. Hypoxia of one kidney or the production of erythropoietin by tumor may be extremely difficult to diagnose. On more than one occasion polycythemia vera, diagnosed on the basis of excluding known cases, has turned out to be due to an abnormality of the hemoglobin molecule impairing O_2 release. Until a time when erythropoietin levels become clinically available and can be monitored in patients with increased hemoglobin levels, there will be certain patients who do not have a definite diagnosis.

PART 3   LABORATORY APPROACH

I.   LABORATORY CAPABILITIES

The availability of hematologic procedures may be discussed at three levels: Emergency procedures are those which must be available at all times. When 24-hour laboratory coverage is not available, the primary care physician must be capable of performing them. Included are the microhematocrit, blood smear (Wright's stain), marrow aspiration for Wright's stained smears, and emergency techniques for the recognizing plasma hemoglobin and methemoglobin. Standard procedures are those which most hematology laboratories can provide on a routine basis and include:

> The hematocrit, hemoglobin and red cell count (cell indices)
> Blood smear preparations (Wright's, reticulocyte and Heinz body stains)
> White blood cell and platelet counts
> Bone marrow aspirate smears for Wright's and iron stains
> Serum iron and iron-binding capacity
> Coombs test (anti-human globulin test)
> Hemoglobin electrophoresis
> Blood volume determinations
> Miscellaneous tests (plasma and urine hemoglobin pigments, etc.)

Finally, there are special laboratory tests which may exceed the capabilities of the standard hematology laboratory but may be essential for establishing a specific diagnosis. Some of these tests must be done locally because of the difficulty in shipping blood without affecting the validity of the test or because the presence of the patient is required. Other procedures may be carried out at distant centralized laboratories.

II.   INTERPRETATION OF LABORATORY RESULTS

Evaluation of any disorder of the erythron usually involves the performance of a number of laboratory measurements in a clinical hematology laboratory. Generally a "routine workup" is performed on every patient. When this demonstrates an abnormality, the physician explores the problem further with an orderly sequence of specific laboratory tests. Such judgment requires an understanding of the technical procedures employed and the limits of accuracy and physiologic variations which surround each measurement. The careful control of each procedure is the responsibility of the laboratory. The expected normal is predicated on the composite distribution of the normal population and any characteristic of the individual which might make him depart from the population mean. Individual procedures have different distribution patterns. The mean and standard deviation is used when a symmetrical distribution is present. The normal male hematocrit value of 47 has a Gaussian (symmetrical) distribution with a standard deviation of $\pm$ 3; that is, 67% of normal males will have hematocrits which range between 44 and 50, while 95% will fall between 41 and 53. Other laboratory measurements may have different patterns of distribution which require other expressions of normalcy. For a very broad distribution of normal values, the expression "range of normal" is frequently used. When abnormal values occur on only one side of a normal distribution, the term "limit of normal" may be employed. Despite these variations in language, the basic decision is always where to make the demarcation between normal and abnormal. This tends to be a probability expression rather than an absolute number (p. 24). Moreover, the large number of modifying factors surrounding any individual case must create a constant uncertainty in interpretating a single value. This represents a major challenge to the physician.

III. GENERAL LABORATORY METHODS

A. Hemoglobin, hematocrit and red cell count (mean cell constants)

The whole blood hemoglobin is measured directly from optical density of oxyhemoglobin when modern automated equipment (Model S Coulter Counter, SMA 7A, Fisher Hem-Alyzer) is employed. In the absence of an automated counter, the hemoglobin level is best determined by diluting a measured volume of mixed venous blood with $K_3Fe(CN_6)$ and KCN solution to form cyanmethemoglobin. The optical density of this pigment is then measured at 540 mμ and compared to a known standard. From a physiologic standpoint the hemoglobin is preferable to other red cell measurements for it provides the most direct indication of the oxygen transport capacity of the blood. However, because of technical advantages, the hematocrit (that volume percent of blood which is red cells) is more often used clinically, especially in emergent situations. The red cell count, when performed through direct enumeration of red cells distributed in a counting chamber by a technician, was previously of limited usefulness because of the error involved. A great advantage of the Coulter Counter is the measurement of a reliable red cell count which permits more extensive use of red cell constants in diagnosis. Erroneously low red cell counts may occasionally result from cold agglutinins or rouleaux formation interfering with individual red cell counting, and erroneously high counts may occur in the presence of a very high white blood cell count, as in a leukemic patient.

The hematocrit is usually determined by spinning a blood-filled capillary tube in a centrifuge. The Model S Coulter Counter provides an indirect measurement of the hematocrit. The diluted blood specimen is passed through an electrical field and the disturbance in electrical conductivity acts as an indicator system. Both the number of erythrocytes per volume of blood and mean cell volume are determined. The percent hematocrit is then calculated by multiplying the mean cell volume by the red cell count. The Model S indirect hematocrit and the centrifugal microhematocrit agree closely through a wide range of abnormalities in cell size and shape. Any unexpected value or major variation between the two should draw attention to the standardization of the Coulter Counter which by the nature of its complexity will more often be in error. Abnormalities of plasma osmolality and electrolyte balance, especially hypo- and hypernatremia, result in a difference between the results of the two techniques. The centrifugal hematocrit measures changes in red cell volume in response to loss or gain of water and electrolytes as they exist in vivo,

whereas the dilution of red cells in normal saline for the Model S Coulter
Counter returns the cells to a normal volume.

Centrifugal Microhematocrit Method

1. Venous blood is drawn from an antecubital vein. Care should be taken
to avoid tourniquet stasis or excessive pain since they will elevate venous
venous hematocrit by as much as 3 or 4 points. The blood is anti- e
coagulated with dry, potassium EDTA (commercial Vacutainers containing
potassium EDTA are available), and then carefully mixed, preferably on
a mechanical rotator.

2. Once adequately mixed, the unmarked end of a plain capillary tube is
placed in the blood without delay and permitted to fill to approximately
3/4 of its length. Tipping toward the horizontal speeds filling. The
tube is then removed from the blood, one end plugged with modeling clay,
wiped clean of excess blood and placed in the centrifuge, clay-filled
end against the rubber gasket. For accuracy, each determination should
be done in duplicate or triplicate.

3. The centrifuge is run for 5 minutes at a set speed (force is
approximately 14,500 x G). This separates red cells from plasma and
leaves a band of white cells and platelets at the interface.

4. The hematocrit is read as that percent of whole venous blood occupied
by red cells. With a constant bore capillary tube this can be done by
obtaining a distance ratio on a microhematocrit reader. The reader is
first set at 100% for the distance from clay-red cell interface to the
plasma meniscus. Then by shifting the ruled scale or etched line to the
red cell-white cell interface the percent hematocrit can be read directly
(white cell volume is considered part of the plasma volume).

For any sample, this measurement should be reproducible at $\pm$ one hematocrit
division. However, additional errors introduced by tourniquet stasis and
physiological plasma volume variations tend to increase this error to $\pm$ 2 when
several venous samples on a single patient are compared. Thus serial hematocrits
may vary between 40 and 44 in a patient without implying a changing situation.

Red cell constants (Wintrobe indices) include the mean cell volume (MCV),
the mean cell hemoglobin (MCH), and the mean cell hemoglobin concentration
(MCHC). The method of calculation and the normal values for these are as
follows:

[handwritten: Macrocytosis = MCV greater th. 98]
[handwritten: Microcytosis = MCV less th. 82.]

$$\text{MCV*} = \frac{\text{hematocrit x 10}}{\text{red cell count x } 10^6} = 90 \pm 8 \ \mu^3$$

$$\text{MCH} = \frac{\text{hemoglobin x 10}}{\text{red cell count x } 10^6} = 30 \pm 3 \ \mu\mu g$$

$$\text{MCHC} = \frac{\text{hemoglobin x 10}}{\text{hematocrit}} \quad \text{or} \quad \frac{\text{MCH}}{\text{MCV}} = 33 \pm 2 \ \text{gm/100 ml red cells}$$

*Measured directly with the Model S Coulter Counter

[handwritten: MCHC = below 28 = iron deficiency anemia (along with microcytic state)]

54

Mean red cell constants are helpful in the initial classification of an anemia and in particular in defining the nature of a maturation abnormality. Certain descriptive terms are used for abnormal values: Macrocytosis when the MCV is greater than 98 and microcytosis when the MCV is less than 82. Artifacts and physiologic changes must be considered before abnormalities in cell development are assumed. The MCV may be high because of an elevated reticulocyte count since young cells are larger than mature cells. Even when the reticulocyte count is not significantly increased, moderate macrocytosis may occur because of increased erythropoietin stimulation. An increase in MCV not explained by methodologic error or by stimulated erythropoiesis indicates a nuclear maturation abnormality. Microcytosis on the other hand implies some abnormality in hemoglobin synthesis. The MCHC is simultaneously decreased by disorders in hemoglobin synthesis, although iron deficiency anemia is the only microcytic state in which the MCHC falls below 28. The MCHC may also be decreased through loss of hemoglobin as with an unstable hemoglobin or with disorders in regulation of cell water which result in overhydration of the cell. An increase in MCHC may be seen in situations of membrane loss (hereditary spherocytosis). The mean corpuscular hemoglobin is most sensitive in detecting a decrease in hemoglobin synthesis within the cell since it compounds the deficits of the decreased MCV and MCHC.

B. Red Cell Morphology

While the cell constants are very useful in detecting general changes in cell size and hemoglobin concentration, they are less sensitive than examination of the blood smear to the presence of a small population of abnormal cells.

The Blood Smear (Wright's Stain)

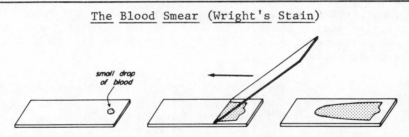

small drop
of blood

1. A small drop of blood, from a fresh EDTA sample or finger stick, is placed on one end of a clean glass slide. Using the edge of a second slide the drop is then drawn the length of the slide with a smooth motion. The thickness of the smear may be varied by the changing of the angle of the applicator slide and the speed of the push.

2. Smears may also be made with coverslips, a technique which offers consistently better red cell morphology. Coverslip smears are made by placing a tiny drop of blood between two coverslips, permitting it to spread and then rapidly pulling them apart. An alternate technique is the preparation of coverslip smears on a smear spinner centrifuge. While this gives more uniform cell distribution, it tends to deform the red cells. The coverslips are then stained and mounted, smear side down, on a glass slide with balsam or methacrylate sealer.

3. The air dried slide is placed in a staining tray and flooded with Wright's stain. After 2-3 minutes, buffer is slowly added to the stain until a green sheen appears on the surface. After 3-5 minutes, the slide is rinsed with tap water and air dried. The optimal timing for the stain and buffer varies for each batch of material and must be determined by trial and error. Once stained, smears can be stored almost indefinitely.

4. Microscopic inspection of slide smears should be limited to the thin portion of the smear where red cells are nearly touching but not overlapping; otherwise, red cell morphology may be distorted. An area should not be considered satisfactory unless the majority of red cells are bi-concave discs.

Red cell morphology provides a wealth of information concerning erythropoiesis, including: 1) evaluation of erythropoietin stimulation, 2) detection of nuclear and cytoplasmic maturation abnormalities, 3) detection of disturbances in marrow architecture and 4) identification of specific disease entities because of unique abnormalities in cell shape. Each smear is inspected under low power, high dry and finally oil immersion, looking for general size and color characteristics of red cells and for cells which show specific abnormalities.

Nuclear maturation abnormalities are characterized by an increase in cell size without a change in the concentration of hemoglobin within the cell. This does not affect all cells uniformly; cell fragments and microcytes are also present as a result of the disorganization of cell replication and maturation an and the subsequent breakage of cells entering circulation. Such an admixture of large and small cells should not lead to misinterpretation of the smear abnormality. The presence of even a rare true macrocyte is sufficient to suggest a nuclear maturation abnormality.

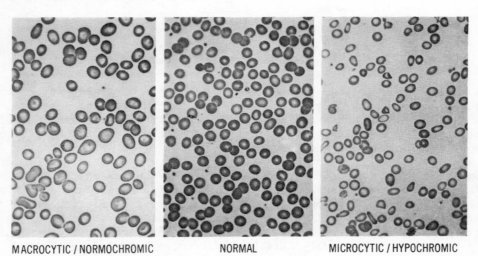

MACROCYTIC / NORMOCHROMIC   NORMAL   MICROCYTIC / HYPOCHROMIC

56

Defects in cytoplasmic maturation (iron deficiency, globin and porphyrin defects) show varying degrees of microcytosis and hypochromia according to their severity. The figure on the preceding page shows a smear in which virtually all cells are both hypochromic and microcytic. On other occasions only a small population of cells may be abnormal. Sometimes cell morphology may seem inconsistent with the mean cell constants. For example, in the anemia of infection, the smear appears to show a slight decrease in cell size with no recognizable change in hemoglobin concentration while the MCV is normal and MCHC slightly decreased. In porphyrin and globin abnormalities (particularly thalassemia), the cells appear very hypochromic and yet the cell indices may show little fall in MCHC. The more severe the maturation defect, the more cell fragmentation (poikilocytosis) is present.

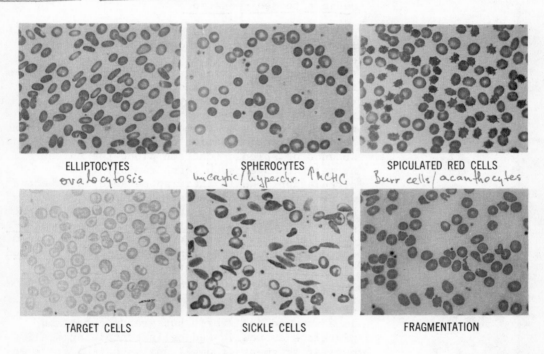

ELLIPTOCYTES
ovalocytosis

SPHEROCYTES
microcytic/hyperchr. ↑MCHC

SPICULATED RED CELLS
Burr cells/acanthocytes

TARGET CELLS

SICKLE CELLS

FRAGMENTATION

In addition to the overall evaluation of cell size and hemoglobin content, characteristic changes in cell shape may provide a direct clue to a specific disease. Most examples of such morphologic trademarks are seen in hemolytic disorders. Elliptocytes (ovalocytes) are easily identified by the oval deformity of the cells; nearly every cell is involved in the patient with hereditary ovalocytosis. Spherocytes are recognized as microcytic/hyperchromic cells (increased MCHC). They result from a loss of red cell membrane and intracellular electrolyte. Spiculated red cells (burr cells, acanthocytes) are also a deformity indicative of red cell membrane damage. Such cells are seen with liver disease, lipid disorders or renal disease. Target cells are the result of an increase in membrane in relation to cell content and represent an increased flattening of the cell. This occurs in many of the hemoglobinopathies including hemoglobin C and S. Targeting is also seen in thalassemia trait, in liver

57

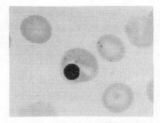

NUCLEATED RED CELL

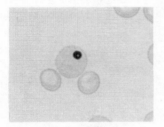

HOWELL JOLLY BODY

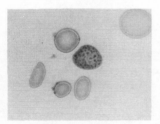

BASOPHILIC STIPPLING

↑Fe
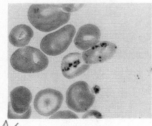

SIDEROCYTE

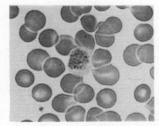

MALARIAL PARASITE

disease (hepatitis, Laennec's cirrhosis and biliary cirrhosis), and to a moderate degree, following splenectomy. With the homozygous form of hemoglobin C and obstructive jaundice, targeting is marked, nearly all cells being involved. Sickle cells are characteristic of the patient with the S hemoglobin gene but their number in the blood smear depends on the number of irreversibly sickled cells in the patient or the degree of deoxygenation of the blood samples used for preparing the smear. Irreversibly sickled cells are the result of membrane damage and are less severely deformed than are sickle cells subject to deoxygenation.

Red cell fragmentation can result from intravascular trauma or damage to newly formed erythrocytes on entrance into circulation (ineffective erythropoiesis). A less severe form of fragmentation (helmet and tear drop cells) is associated with the removal of a Heinz body from the red cell. Nucleated red cells, usually late normoblasts, but sometimes earlier red cell forms, indicate disorganization of red cell delivery and/or absence of splenic function since the spleen normally removes such forms rapidly from circulation. While their appearance is expected whenever erythropoietin stimulation is extremely high (severe hemolytic and maturation defect anemias anemias), the presence of circulating nucleated red cells in a patient with a hypoproliferative anemia suggests marrow damage and in particular invasion of the marrow by metastatic tumor, leukemia or fibrous tissue. This situation is often referred to as a myelophthisic blood picture, involving the presence in the circulating blood not only of immature red cell forms but granulocytes and platelets as well. Red cells containing small nuclear fragments (Howell Jolly bodies) are some- times seen in patients with a poorly functioning or absent spleen. In contrast to the nucleated red cell, they do not imply marrow structural damage. Basophilic stippling may be seen in occasional red cells on the normal smear, representing a reticulocyte whose basophilia is punctate rather than diffuse. Heavier stippling is seen with marrow stromal abnormalities and with increased erythropoietin stimulation. The presence of very heavy stippling should always raise the consideration of lead poisoning. A number of small irregular granules in a red cell should suggest the presence of iron-laden mitochondria (siderocytes).

This is easily confirmed with an iron stain of the blood smear. In the presence of fever and a hemolytic anemia, a careful search should be made for intracellular malarial parasites. Thick preparations with special staining (Wright-Giemsa) are usually required to assist in the diagnosis. The presence of the various abnormal red cell forms mentioned may be difficult to recognize because of the small number of such forms present. Since they are usually lighter than the normal cells, centrifugation is often employed (buffy coat preparation) to assist in their detection.

C. Measurements of Production and Maturation

In most clinical situations, the level of marrow production and the characteristics of cell maturation and destruction are defined using the reticulocyte count and bone marrow aspirate.

Reticulocyte Count

1. EDTA anticoagulated blood is mixed with a 0.5% solution of new methylene blue (color index no. 52030) in equal amounts – two drops of blood added to two drops of new methylene blue solution.

2. After 10-15 minutes, the tube is shaken and coverslip smears are prepared using a small drop of the mixture. The coverslips are permitted to air dry for at least 10 minutes before counterstaining. It is preferable to use the blood smear centrifuge when available to prepare reticulocyte smears. This technique guarantees a more uniform distribution of reticulocytes and reduces the error of the method.

3. The dry smears are fixed with 95% methanol, counterstained with Wright's stain and mounted on a large glass slide with methacrylate sealer.

4. Reticulocytes are those cells containing dark blue staining material in granules or strands. Routinely the number of reticulocytes seen while counting 1000 red cells in consecutive high power fields is sufficient for determining the reticulocyte percentage. For high reticulocyte counts this is quite accurate. The standard error of the method ($\pm$ 2 S.E.) for a reticulocyte count of 15.0% is $\pm$ 2.3; with a count of 1.0% the limits are 0.4 to 1.6. For accurate determinations at reticulocyte counts of less than 5%, 2000 or more cells must be counted.

In the basal state, a normal individual replaces approximately 1% of his circulating red cells each day. This results in a 1.0% reticulocyte count inasmuch as the small amount of stainable RNA in these cells is lost over a 24-27 hour period. (Because of the counting error at this low level, the normal reticulocyte percentage will appear to range between 0.5 and 1.5%.) As long as the hematocrit and level of erythropoietin stimulation are normal, this observed reticulocyte percentage may also be considered an index of production – normal reticulocyte production index = 1.

With anemia, the observed reticulocyte percentage reflects not only the level of marrow production but also a decline in the total number of adult cells diluting each day's reticulocyte production. Thus, an individual whose rate of production is unchanged but whose hematocrit has fallen to 23 from 46% will have an observed reticulocyte percentage of 2 but a normal production index. In this situation a normal number of reticulocytes are diluted by only half the normal number of circulating adult cells, effectively doubling the percentage count. Therefore, with a lower than normal hematocrit, the reticulocyte count must be first corrected to a hematocrit of 45 before calculating the production index.

A further correction is required when erythropoietin stimulation results in premature delivery of marrow reticulocytes to circulation (reticulocyte "shift,") since these young reticulocytes require 2-3 days to lose their reticulum. The Wright's stained smear is carefully inspected for the presence of pale blue macrocytes or "shift" cells. When these are easily visible the reticulocyte count is further corrected using a factor of two or according to the severity of the anemia. As discussed on page 18, there is a progressive lengthening of the reticulocyte maturation time with increasing anemia. An example of the full calculation is as follows:

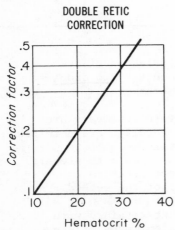

DOUBLE RETIC CORRECTION

Correction factor

Hematocrit %

If a patient has a 9% reticulocyte count, a hematocrit of 25%, and easily visible "shift" cells on smear, his production index is obtained using both corrections –

$$\text{Reticulocyte production index} = \frac{9\% \times \frac{25}{45} \text{ (hematocrit correction)}}{2.0 \text{ (maturation time correction)}} = 2.5$$

The reticulocyte production index calculated in this fashion is an approximate measure of effective red cell production. A normal individual's erythroid marrow is not a static organ. It responds to anemia by rapid proliferation and a 2-5 fold increase in red cell production. Thus, a significant abnormality or marrow function because of marrow damage, erythropoietin suppression, deficient iron supply, or maturation disorder may be suspected whenever there is a less than normal marrow response (p. 19). Values greater than 3 are characteristic of hemolytic anemias where the iron from greatly increased red cell destruction permits high levels of marrow production.

In most situations, the reticulocyte index is sufficient to separate disorders of marrow proliferation and maturation from hemolytic anemias. Further help in the separation of proliferative from maturation defects is obtained from a simultaneous evaluation of the marrow E/G ratio. With hypoproliferative and hemolytic anemias, the marrow E/G ratio decreases or increases in parallel with the reticulocyte response. On the other hand, disorders of nuclear or cytoplasmic maturation characteristically show a discrepancy between the number of marrow normoblasts and the reticulocyte count so that erythroid hyperplasia (high E/G ratio) is not reflected in a proportionate increase of the reticulocyte index.

Bone Marrow Aspirate

1. Employing a special, heavy-walled bone marrow needle, the marrow cavity is entered and small amounts of marrow aspirated. The puncture is best performed along the posterior superior iliac crest, the anterior iliac crest, or the sternum. After a full skin prep, the skin and periosteum are infiltrated with 1 or 2% procaine. The marrow needle is then worked through the outer table of bone with a slight twisting motion. Entry into the marrow is marked by a sudden loss of resistance and momentary pain from endosteal nerve fibers.

2. A first drop of marrow is removed with a small syringe (such as a tuberculin syringe) and touch smears made by an assistant. Next, about 2 ml of marrow is aspirated with a syringe containing 2 ml of EDTA solution. This is mixed and expelled onto a watch glass.

3. Using a capillary tube, 4-5 marrow particles are picked up from this solution, placed on a coverslip and smeared after excess blood has been removed. At least a dozen smears should be made.

4. The smears are fixed with 95% methanol and then stained with Wright's stain. Once air dried they are mounted with methacrylate. The optimal staining time will vary for each batch of stain and will be longer than the time used for peripheral smears. Heavy smears will be more satisfactory if counterstained with Giemsa.

Whenever anemia is due to a production defect whose nature is unclear, a bone marrow aspirate is indicated. Marrow smears are inspected under low power and oil immersion for the following:

a) Adequacy of specimen
b) Megakaryocyte number and type
c) Abnormal cells - tumor cells, plasma cells, etc.
d) Visual estimate of the normoblast granulocyte (E/G) ratio
e) Abnormal maturation patterns -
    red cells - nuclear or cytoplasmic maturation defect
    white cells - megaloblastosis; leukemia; reduction in the marrow
      granulocyte reserve

Once the adequacy of the specimen is confirmed, the E/G ratio is approximated by scanning a number of cellular fields under oil immersion and estimating the relative number of immature erythroid cells. Laborious counting of a small area of cellular elements does not improve the accuracy of the ratio, since the distribution of red cell and granulocyte elements on smears of aspirated marrow is not random. With a little practice, it is not difficult to distinguish the normal E/G ratio of 1:2 to 1:3 from that of a stimulated marrow, for the E/G ratio should increase to better than 1:1 within five days of the onset of even a mild anemia. Any response which falls short of this ratio indicates a hypoproliferative defect, while increased E/G ratios are common to both hemolytic and maturation abnormalities. Qualitative changes in marrow cells (megaloblastic, sideroblastic or leukemic transformations) provide additional help in diagnosing the marrow abnormality. Interpretation of the E/G ratio is only valid when the granulocyte mass is normal. This is usually evaluated from the number of circulating normal granulocytes. In the presence of altered granulocyte proliferation or infiltration of the marrow with tumor cells, little idea of erythroid proliferation can be derived from the aspirate. Obviously, the same is true when a "dry tap" or inadequate specimen is obtained. A marrow biopsy and section provides more useful information concerning overall cellularity. Moreover, in the more perplexing patient, where a quantitative measurement of erythroid marrow activity is required, radioiron kinetic studies (plasma iron turnover and ferrokinetics with organ counting) may be employed.

Indirect measurements of overall red cell turnover which are often available in the routine laboratory data base of the hospitalized patient are the bilirubin and lactic dehydrogenase (LDH). The normal concentration of <u>bilirubin</u> in plasma is between .4 and .9 mg%. Unusually low values are found with hypoproliferative and hemorrhagic anemias, while increases of from 1 to 2 mg% accompany hemolytic anemias or maturation disorders with marked ineffective erythropoiesis. Since increased red cell turnover should only result in a small increase in the indirect indirect fraction (unconjugated bilirubin), major elevations in total bilirubin or a large direct fraction should implicate liver disease (rarely there is a congenital defect in bilirubin conjugation). <u>LDH</u> elevation accompanies damage to a variety of tissues, particularly the liver. Increased serum levels are also seen in the hemolytic anemias, especially with intravascular hemolysis where the enzyme is cleared more slowly than hemoglobin. In the usual patient with a hemolytic anemia, LDH concentration ranges between 200 and 800 units/ml. With megaloblastic anemias, for reasons which are not entirely clear, marked elevations to several thousand units are found and there is a reversal of the LDH isozyme pattern (LDH 1 exceeds LDH 2 activity).

D. Measurements of Iron Supply

The examination of iron delivery and storage is important to the differential diagnosis of both maturation and hypoproliferative disorders. Included are measurements of the serum iron (SI) and total iron-binding capacity (TIBC), an inspection of marrow stroma particles for stainable reticuloendothelial stores and a careful search for the type and number of marrow sideroblasts. In some situations, a red cell protoporphyrin level may be helpful.

<u>Serum Iron and TIBC Methods</u> (<u>82</u>)

1. Most macroassays require at least 10 ml of venous blood, drawn with a plastic syringe or directly into an iron-free vacutainer tube. Once the cells are separated, samples may be stored for at least five days at 4°C without loss of accuracy. To measure iron content, the serum is acidified, protein precipitated and a chromagen solution bathophenanthroline sulfonate added. The optical density of the iron-chromagen can then be measured.

---

2. The amount of transferrin protein is measured as the total iron
binding capacity (TIBC). Ferric chloride solution is added to serum,
followed by magnesium carbonate powder in order to absorb excess iron not
bound to transferrin. After this, the tube is centrifuged and the supernatant treated as for the measurement of the serum iron. As an
alternative technique, the ferric chloride solution can be labeled with
radioiron and the iron binding capacity determined from the radioactivity
remaining in the supernatant after magnesium carbonate absorption.

The serum iron method described above is not affected by hemolysis
(hemoglobin iron) but does measure 10-30% of circulating iron dextran (Imferon).
Thus, in patients receiving parenteral iron, the interpretation of the serum iron
may be invalidated for several weeks. A similar proportion of circulating
ferritin may be measured and occasionally, this may contribute significantly to
the serum iron concentration. The wide range of normal serum iron values (mean
110 µg/100 ml; range 70-150) is in part due to the diurnal cycling of plasma
iron. Since the high point is usually in the morning and the most common
diagnostic problem is the detection of
iron-deficiency, a fasting morning
sample is preferable. Iron-deficient
erythropoiesis is considered to exist
whenever the transferrin saturation
falls to 15% or less. At the same
time, attention should be paid to the
TIBC, since it helps separate iron-
deficient patients without iron stores
from those individuals who develop
internal iron blockade secondary to
inflammation. In contrast to the higher
than normal TIBC of absolute iron
deficiency, the patient with
inflammation has a decreased transferrin
level. Other abnormal patterns of
iron and TIBC are shown in the
accompanying figure. With marrow
damage, ineffective erythropoiesis or

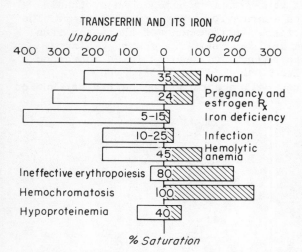

parenchymal iron overload, the serum iron tends to rise, leading to full
saturation of the TIBC in more severe cases. The TIBC will also change in
response to altered protein or hormonal balance. However, because of
corresponding changes in the plasma iron, the percent saturation is still valid.

Iron Stain of the Marrow (83)

1. Coverslip smears of marrow particles are placed in Coplin jars and
fixed in absolute methanol for 4-24 hours. An equal part mixture of 2%
HCl and 2% potassium ferrocyanide is preheated for 1-2 minutes at 56°C;
the fixed smears are then incubated in this stain for 10 minutes at 56°C.

2. To stop the staining reaction, the smears are immediately washed in
running tap water for at least 20 minutes. Then they are counterstained
with 0.1% safranin for 10 seconds and mounted with methacrylate.

Iron stores appear as agglomerates and fine, single granules of blue-staining material in the cytoplasm of the reticuloendothelial cells. Hemosiderin particles are also visible as golden-brown granules in the unstained preparation. Preferably both types of preparation should be used, but the most important feature is the presence of marrow particles of adequate size. With as little as 100 mg of body iron stores, iron should be visible on careful inspection, making thi this an extremely reliable method for detecting absolute iron store deficiency. Normal iron stores (500-1500 mg of mobilizable iron) are easily visible (as 2 to 3+ stores on a scale of 0 to 6+), while iron overload can result in dense blue-staining visible on gross inspection of the slide. This assessment can be of prime value in distinguishing the absolute iron-deficient patient (absent iron stores) from the internal iron blockade of inflammatory states, where iron stores are present but mobilization from the reticuloendothelial cell is impaired. Moreover, the patient with chronic inflammation frequently has very large chunky granules within his RE cells.

The presence of visible iron granules in red cell precursors (sideroblasts) reflects both the level of iron supply and the status of hemoglobin synthesis. In normal individuals 30-60% of normoblasts contain 1-4 tiny iron granules. The percentage of these sideroblasts falls to less than 10 whenever the serum iron falls, with either true iron deficiency or inflammation. By contrast, intra-cellular defects of iron incorporation into hemoglobin results in an increased percentage of sideroblasts and number of iron granules per cell. The significance of iron granules within the red cell according to their distribution has been previously discussed (p. 4).

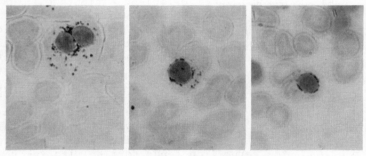

ABNORMAL AND RING SIDEROBLASTS

Red cell protoporphyrin is also of value in detecting iron-deficient erythropoiesis. The protoporphyrin level increases to values above 100 μg/100 ml of red cells as iron delivery falls below normal; increases also rarely occur with abnormalities in porphyrin synthesis.

Measurement of Red Cell Protoporphyrin (43)

Fresh or frozen whole blood is treated with acetone: ethyl acetate and then extracted with two volumes of formic acid: ether. After removal of precipitated red cell stroma, the formic acid: ether supernatant is shaken vigorously with 1.5 N HCl and the absorbance of the HCl-protoporphyrin solution measured.

E. Blood Volume Measurements

In situations of rapidly changing fluid balance or blood volume loss and replacement, measurements of plasma volume and red cell mass can be important. Moreover, these techniques are often needed for the differential diagnosis of polycythemia. For direct measurements of the red cell mass and plasma volume either radiolabeled red cells or I^{131} albumin are used.

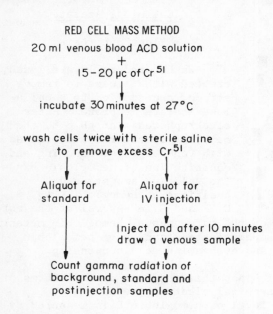

RED CELL MASS METHOD
20 ml venous blood ACD solution
+
15–20 μc of Cr^{51}

incubate 30 minutes at 27°C

wash cells twice with sterile saline to remove excess Cr^{51}

Aliquot for standard

Aliquot for IV injection

Inject and after 10 minutes draw a venous sample

Count gamma radiation of background, standard and postinjection samples

Cr^{51} avidly binds to the hemoglobin molecule of the adult red cell and only a small sample of the patient's blood is required for labeling. By measuring the radioactivity of the injected Cr^{51}-tagged cells and a venous blood sample after intravenous mixing, the red cell mass (ml) is obtained from the calculation:

$$\frac{\text{Total counts injected}}{\text{counts/ml venous blood}} \times \text{hematocrit}$$

Accurate plasma volume measurement is complicated by the tendency of albumin

PLASMA VOLUME METHOD
RISA – radioiodinated human serum albumin
5–10 μc

Standard aliquot or count rate of entire solution

Aliquot for IV injection

Inject and draw 1–4 venous samples (after 10 minutes)

Count gamma radiation of background, standard and postinjection samples

to leak out of the intravascular space. In most clinical situations, this leak can be estimated as 5% in the first 10–20 minutes and thus compensated for by using the factor 1.05. Plasma volume (ml) is obtained from the calculation:

$$\frac{\text{Total counts injected}}{\text{counts/ml plasma} \times 1.05} \times (100-\text{hct})$$

When both the red cell mass and plasma volume are measured, the total blood volume is the simple sum. From either measurement the total blood volume may be calculated using a correction factor to derive the total body hematocrit from the measured venous hematocrit (total body hematocrit = venous hematocrit x 0.91). For clinical purposes, the measured volumes are expressed according to body weight (ml/kg), though it is recognized that major deviations from lean body mass, obesity or severe starvation, will lead to a major error. Commonly used normal values for males in ml/kg are: red cell mass = 30 ± 3 and plasma volume = 40 ± 4. Measurements in females show a slightly smaller red cell mass (25 ml/kg), but a similar plasma volume.

F. Hemoglobin Stability and Electrophoretic Migration

When there is a possibility of an abnormal hemoglobin or a defect in globin production, tests of hemoglobin pH stability and electrophoretic mobility are performed. Common screening tests include cellulose acetate electrophoresis, alkali denaturation, and a sickle cell screen.

CELLULOSE ACETATE ELECTROPHORESIS

DISEASE	ORIGIN →	A_2	C	S	F	A
Normal					▮	▇
Sickle cell trait				▮		▇
Sickle cell disease				▇	▮	
Sickle-C			▮	▇		
C-trait			▮			▇
Thalassemia major					▇	▮
Thalassemia minor					▮	▇
Sickle-thalassemia				▮	▮	▮

Cellulose Acetate Electrophoresis

Washed red cells are lysed, treated with toluene to remove stroma, and applied to a cellulose acetate membrane. After electrophoresis at pH 8.8, the membrane is cleared and stained with Ponceau S for scanning and quantitation of hemoglobin bands. The relative amounts and positions of hemoglobins A_2, S, C, F and A in several of the more common hemoglobinopathies are shown. Some of the more unusual hemoglobin mutants may only be identified by performing more sophisticated studies of hemoglobin mobility, heat stability, O_2 dissociation, and even amino acid sequencing.

Accurate identification of many hemoglobinopathies and the several forms of α and β thalassemia may require agar or starch gel electrophoresis and quantitation of A_2 and F hemoglobins. The level of hemoglobin F is measured by taking advantage of its greater resistance to precipitation at alkaline pH. Red cell hemolysate is briefly exposed to a dilute solution of potassium hydroxide and the precipitable hemoglobin removed by $(NH_4)_2SO_4$ precipitation and filtration. The amount of hemoglobin F remaining in the supernatant is then measured colorimetrically (84). Hemoglobin S is identified by its unique ability to form tactoids and thereby deform red cell shape on deoxygenation. This physical property is the basis of a number of rapid screening tests, including the metabisulfite preparation and the solubility test (85). These methods must be considered inferior to the cellulose acetate electrophoresis technique, however, since they do not measure the amount of S hemoglobin or detect the presence of other abnormal hemoglobins (86).

IV. SPECIAL LABORATORY METHODS

A. Measurements of Folate and Vitamin B_{12} Supply

Evaluation of a nuclear maturation defect includes measurements of plasma vitamin levels, absorption tests and at times the patient's response to specific therapy. The serum vitamin B_{12} level may be measured by microbiological assay or by isotope dilution. Both Euglena gracilis and Lactobacillus leichmanii require vitamin B_{12} for growth and may be used for the microbiological procedure. The isotope dilution technique measures the serum B_{12} level according to its ability to compete with a known amount of $Co^{57}B_{12}$ for a specific binding protein, such as intrinsic factor (87,88). Normal individuals have serum vitamin B_{12} levels of 200 $\mu\mu g/ml$ or more; deficiency should be suspected when values fall below this level. In the presence of abnormal binding proteins, especially with severe liver disease, vitamin B_{12} delivery may be deficient despite an apparent normal serum level. Vitamin B_{12} deficiency may also be detected by assay of urine for its content of <u>methylmalonic acid</u> (89,90). An abnormal result is specific for B_{12} deficiency. A 24-hour urine specimen is collected under toluene and stored at $-15^{o}C$ until assay. Aliquots are acidified, extracted with ether and the extract assayed by thin layer or two dimensional paper chromatography. Normal individuals excrete less than 10 mg/day while individuals with vitamin B_{12} deficiency can have several hundred milligrams in a 24-hour urine specimen. For reasons which are unclear, an occasional patient with vitamin B_{12} deficiency may show normal methylmalonic acid excretion.

Once vitamin B_{12} deficiency has been demonstrated, it is necessary to identify its cause. The Schilling test (with and without intrinsic factor) and the gastric free acid determination are most commonly employed.

<u>Schilling Test (91)</u>

Cobalt[57]-labeled vitamin B_{12} is given in liquid or capsule form to the fasting patient. A 20 ml venous blood sample is drawn at the time of administration for a background count. One hour later, 1000 μg of vitamin B_{12} is injected intramuscularly and a 24-hour urine collection started. Eight hours after isotope administration, a second 20 ml venous sample is drawn. The plasma radioactivity is then determined and compared to a standard prepared from the orally administered $Co^{57}B_{12}$. An aliquot of the 24-hour urine may also be counted. The amount of vitamin B_{12} absorbed is calculated both as the amount circulating in plasma at 8 hours and the percent appearing in the urine after the flushing dose of 1000 μg. In the normal individual the 8 hour plasma level is greater than 0.18% of the dose/1% body weight and the 24-hour urinary excretion is greater than 7%.

The cause of an abnormal value is further studied to differentiate between intrinsic factor deficiency and a defect in ileal absorption. This is accomplished by repeating the Schilling test with exogenous intrinsic factor. Co^{57}-labeled B_{12} is given orally together with a capsule of desiccated pig intrinsic factor or 100 ml of fresh normal human gastric juice. The procedure is then identical to the Schilling test. Correction of vitamin B_{12} absorption to normal with intrinsic factor usually indicates vitamin B_{12} malabsorption due to intrinsic factor deficiency. Other causes, i.e. bacterial overgrowth, parasitic infestation, small bowel tumor or resections, etc., should not correct. Deficiency of intrinsic factor may also be inferred from the absence of gastric free acid after histamine stimulation. The simplest test employs a commercially available cation exchange resin, Diagnex Blue. When histalog stimulation is used with this material, there are only 5% false negatives and probably no false positive results. The procedure is described in full on the Diagnex Blue kit. Still considered somewhat more reliable, however, is the intragastric acid determination by intubation.

```
                    Gastric Free Acid Method (92)

1.  A nasogastric tube is passed in the morning while fasting.  Stomach
contents are aspirated and tested for free acid with a pH meter or at the
bedside with Topfer's reagent, 3 drops added to 10-20 ml of gastric
juice.  The color changes from yellow to red at pH 3.0, indicating free
acid.

2.  If negative, the patient is given one ml of "histalog" (a histamine
analog) subcutaneously and a second aspiration done after 30-40 minutes.
Continued achlorohydria, pH greater than 3.5 indicates parietal cell
atrophy and intrinsic factor lack.  A low pH associated with a small
volume of gastric secretion should be studied further by measurement of
total titratable acidity.
```

Serum folic acid levels are measured by a microbiological assay employing
Lactobacillus casei or with an isotope dilution technique employing milk protein
as a binder (93). To ensure an accurate measurement, it is essential that
hemolysis be kept at a minimum when the serum sample is obtained. Red cells
contain large amounts of mono- and polyglutamates, so that even minor amounts of
hemolysis can falsely elevate the serum level. To avoid falsely low values, it
is important that the serum be assayed soon after drawing since folic acid can
deteriorate with storage or travel. Also, the test should not be performed
while a patient is on antibiotics, since even small amounts in the serum may
inhibit bacterial growth.

B. Hemolytic Procedures

Destruction Measurements: Direct measurements of red cell destruction (the
number of cells destroyed per day or the life span of individual red cells) are
far less accurate and more difficult to perform than production measurements.
Estimating the destruction index from the production index and changes in the
hematocrit over a period of several days remains the most applicable technique
for patient evaluation. When the patient's hematocrit has been measured
repeatedly over a 5-10 day period, a red cell destruction index may be
approximated from the production index and the tendency for the hematocrit to
rise or fall. For example, if the hematocrit falls while the production index is
5 times normal, it follows that destruction index must be greater than 5 times
normal.

Confusion may arise concerning the terms "destruction rate," which relates
to the life span of the red cell, and "destruction index," which refers to the
total number of cells being destroyed each day. When analyzing the destruction
pattern of an anemia, the life span of the circulating red cells (destruction
rate) and the number of cells dying each day (destruction index) are not
necessarily the same. For example, a patient with a normal production index
(index = 1) and a stable hematocrit of 23% destroys a normal number of cells each
day but the life span of his cells is one-half normal (about 50-60 days) instead
of the normal 100-120 days. A simple formula may be set up for conversion from
life span to destruction index. (This should be applied only to situations
where the hematocrit is stable).

$$\text{Destruction index} = \frac{60 \ (\text{normal mean cell life-span})}{\text{patient's mean cell life-span (days)}} \ x \ \frac{\text{patient's hematocrit}}{45}$$

Direct measurements of the red cell destruction rate (life-span) may be accomplished in man by determining the disappearance rate of his own red cells labeled with either Cr^{51} or DFP^{32} isotope. In the normal individual any venous blood sample represents a random selection of cells of all ages, from 1-120 days.

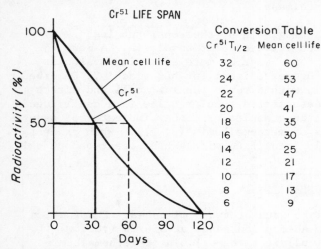

Cr^{51} LIFE SPAN

Mean cell life

Cr^{51}

Radioactivity (%)

Days

Conversion Table

$Cr^{51}T_{1/2}$	Mean cell life
32	60
24	53
22	47
20	41
18	35
16	30
14	25
12	21
10	17
8	13
6	9

Once labeled, these randomly distributed cells disappear in a linear fashion over the next 120 days with 50% gone (T 1/2) at 60 days. In the case of DFP^{32}-labeled cells, this is true. However, when Cr^{51} is used, there is the complicating factor of Cr^{51} elution from cells prior to death. This results in an apparent shortening of the normal T 1/2 to 32 days. The <u>expected</u> curve for a random age population and the actual disappearance curve of the Cr^{51} isotope are compared in the figure. A conversion table to correct for the elution phenomenon when survival is shortened accompanies the graph. Despite its simplicity, the Cr^{51} life-span is infrequently employed in clinical evaluations. Technical errors, unpredictable Cr^{51} elution rates and the long delay before useful data are obtained tend to decrease its value. Any excessive blood loss during the test tends to falsely shorten the T 1/2. If the initial labeled population does not represent random ages, but is skewed by a large number of younger, recently produced cells, the apparent T 1/2 may actually be longer than 30 days. The major usefulness of the technique is to distinguish between extracellular and intracellular mechanisms of cell destruction (p. 45) and to study the relative importance or spleen and liver uptake in a red cell destructive process.

1. Intravascular Hemolysis

It is often of diagnostic importance to identify the type of hemolysis. Especially in acute hemolytic anemias, the distinction between intravascular and extravascular hemolysis can be a major step toward diagnosis. With significant <u>intravascular</u> hemolysis, as with a mismatched transfusion, thermal burn or <u>Clostridium welchii</u> lysin, the findings depend on the time elapsed since the event. During or immediately thereafter, cell fragmentation and/or spherocyte formation may be seen on smear along with hemoglobinemia and hemoglobinuria. If a heparinized venous blood sample is drawn, centrifuged and the plasma inspected for hemolysis, intravascular lysis of 5-10 ml or more of packed red cells should be visible (a plasma hemoglobin concentration of greater than 50 mg%). With reasonable care, hemolysis secondary to blood drawing and processing should not exceed 30 mg% plasma hemoglobin.

Hemoglobinuria may be detected visually in a centrifued urine specimen or with the commercial "Occultest" tablet. To distinguish true hemoglobinuria from hypotonic lysis of hematuric red cells, a simultaneous plasma sample should always be inspected. A positive "Occultest" without obvious hemoglobinemia is almost certainly due to either hematuria or myoglobinuria. The Occultest tablet available for identifying hemoglobinuria must never be used to detect hemoglobinemia since positive reactions will occur with as little as 1 mg%, a level present in all normal plasma specimens.

Because of active resorption of hemoglobin by the renal tubules, hemoglobinuria is seen only with severe intravascular hemolysis. A more sensitive test which may be positive for a week or more after intravascular hemolysis is the examination of spun urine sediment for hemosiderin. Resorbed hemoglobin is converted to hemosiderin within renal tubular cells and direct examination or an iron stain or the desquamated tubular cells in a centrifuged urine sediment will show the hemosiderin granules. Another indicator of severe hemolysis is the appearance in plasma of methemalbumin (p. 11). When present in appreciable amounts, it may be rapidly identified with a hand spectroscope using the Schumm Test.

Schumm Test

1. Two ml of plasma is pipetted into each of two 5 ml tubes. Examination with a hand spectroscope will show absorption bands at 576 mμ (yellow) if hemoglobin is present and 630 mμ (red) if methemoglobin or methemalbumin is present, although the latter band may be weak.

2. To one tube, 0.2 ml of concentrated ammonium sulfide is added after layering the plasma with ether. If methemalbumin is present, the 630 mμ (red) band will disappear and a dense 558 mμ (green) band will appear. The tube should be examined immediately since on standing the sulfide will tend to produce sulfhemoglobin with an absorption band at 618 mμ.

Paroxysmal nocturnal hemoglobinuria (PNH) may be suspected in individuals with a severe hemolytic or hypoplastic anemia and associated hemosiderinuria. Screening tests for PNH involve demonstrating the tendency of the patient's cells to hemolyze in solutions of low ionic strength in the presence of complement.

Sucrose Screening Test (PNH) (94)

1. A 50% saline suspension of patient and control cells is prepared from red cells collected in oxalate or citrate and washed three times in saline.

2. Fresh compatible serum or AB serum, frozen at -70°C, is then mixed with the cell suspension (.05 ml serum with 0.1 ml cell suspension). This is added to 0.85 ml of freshly prepared sucrose solution (10 gm sucrose in 100 ml distilled water).

3. After mixing, the tube is centrifuged and examined for gross hemolysis.

---

2. Extravascular Hemolysis

Extravascular or reticuloendothelial hemolysis is typical of the majority of hemolytic disorders, including defects in the membrane, in aerobic or anaerobic metabolism, in hemoglobin stability, or with reticuloendothelial disease. Evaluation of an extravascular hemolytic process involves severeal screening tests and a number of sophisticated techniques to pinpoint the defect. Especially in the area of congenital intracellular defects, the specialized hematology laboratory will be needed.

Considering the frequency of various hemolytic disorders and the availability of laboratory techniques, an extravascular hemolytic process is best approached in the following sequence:

1. Careful review of the peripheral blood smear for evidence of a characteristic shape abnormality - spherocytosis, sickle cells, etc., (p. 57).

2. Search for an autoimmune process - Coombs test, cold agglutinins, LE prep, ANF, etc.

3. Heinz body preparation and G6PD screen.

4. Hemoglobin electrophoresis on several different media - cellulose acetate, starch gel, agar gel, etc.

5. Studies of osmotic fragility and autohemolysis as general tests of membrane function and intracellular metabolic pathways.

6. Determination of heat stability of hemoglobin.

7. Determination of other enzyme activities, levels of ATP, 2,3-DPG or other glycolytic intermediates.

a. Autoimmune Disease

The interaction of membrane antigen and circulating antibody can result in either intravascular lysis and/or agglutination of cells or membrane coating sufficient to cause early reticuloendothelial destruction. Agglutination by antibodies of the IgM class may be grossly visible on inspection of an anticoagulated venous sample. For less obvious antibodies, the Coombs test is employed. Specific characteristics of the antibody type (p. 42) can be important both for diagnosis and management.

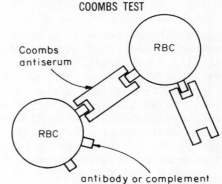

COOMBS TEST

The <u>Coombs test</u> employs an antiserum containing antibodies directed against human IgG and complement so as to act as an agglutinating bridge between antibody or complement-coated red cells. The <u>direct</u>

71

Coombs test looks for antibody attached to circulating red cells, while the indirect Coombs test detects antibodies in the patient's plasma. By using specific antisera (anti-IgG or anti-complement) this test may be used to classify the human antibodies. In some cases, specificity of the plasma antibodies may be further determined by performing the indirect Coombs test against a panel of human red cells whose membrane antigens are known.

Traditionally, IgM cold reacting autoantibodies have been measured in hospital laboratories by the cold agglutinin test. This is in essence a titration of antibodies showing high degrees of cold reactivity for the patient's or group O red cells. Patients with significant autohemolysis have titers exceeding 1:1000. The direct Coombs test in these patients is either negative or weakly positive.

Cold Agglutinins

Venous blood is collected in a warm syringe and clotted at 37°C. The serum is separated. Washed group O red cells are used to make a 1% suspension in saline. Serial saline dilutions of the serum are made from 1:2 to 1:65,000. To 0.5 ml of these dilutions, 0.5 ml of the 1% red cell suspension is added, incubated for 2 hours at room temperature and then read for agglutination. They are then placed in the refrigerator (4°C) overnight to be read while cold.

---

b. Membrane Defects

The most common abnormality of the red cell membrane is hereditary spherocytosis. While recognition is not always easy because of variability of genetic expression, the incubated osmotic fragility and autohemolysis tests are commonly used to screen for this condition.

Autohemolysis Test

Venous blood is defibrinated and transferred into sterile capped tubes. Glucose is added to duplicate tubes. After 24 hours of incubation at 37°C, all tubes are gently mixed. At 48 hours they are again mixed, a sample removed for hematocrit and hemoglobin determination and the tubes centrifuged. A hemoglobin determination is then carried out on the serum.

Normal blood shows 2-5% hemolysis without glucose, reduced to 0-1% when glucose is added. Patients with hereditary spherocytosis or elliptocytosis classically demonstrate 4-50% hemolysis without glucose but only 1-2% with glucose. As with the incubated osmotic fragility, an autoimmune hemolytic anemia with spherocytes may mimic the findings of hereditary spherocytosis. In contrast, metabolic defects (pyruvate kinase deficiency, etc.) fail to show correction of hemolysis with glucose but may demonstrate less hemolysis following addition of ATP. While the autohemolysis test is a valuable screening procedure, the frequency of both false negatives and the additional disorders which have an associated abnormal test reduce its specificity.

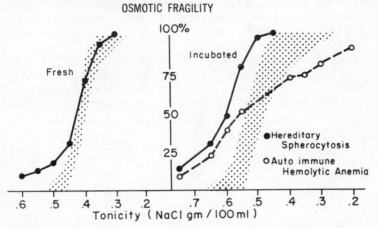

OSMOTIC FRAGILITY

      In hereditary spherocytosis there is a variable increase in osmotic
fragility which should become more obvious after incubation. In autoimmune
hemolytic anemias there may also be a population of spherocytic cells with
increased fragility, but the curve tends to cross over due to a population of
more resistant cells.

      c.   Intracellular Metabolic Defects

      A number of screening procedures and specific tests of enzyme function are
available to help identify defects in cell metabolism and hemoglobin stability.
While most of these require the expertise of the research laboratory, the Heinz
body preparation, alcohol denaturation test for unstable hemoglobins, and G6PD
and pyruvate kinase enzyme spot tests may be used for screening purposes.

      This test is used to detect the presence of Heinz bodies, small particles
of precipitated hemoglobin, in circulating red cells as a part of an ongoing

hemolytic process. Even a small number of Heinz bodies in a few red cells is significant. A more elaborate test involving incubation with acetylphenyl-hydrazine may be useful as provocative screen for G6PD deficiency, other abnormalities in the shunt pathway or an unstable hemoglobin (95).

Isopropanol Denaturation Test (96)

A stroma-free hemolysate is prepared from fresh blood, taking care to avoid extraction of unstable hemoglobins. 0.2 ml of the hemolysate is added to a 17% (by volume) solution of buffered isopropanol. After incubation at 37°C for 5 minutes the solution is examined for turbidity.

The appearance of a flocculent precipitate suggests an unstable hemoglobin and should stimulate additional studies (hemoglobin electrophoresis, brilliant cresyl blue incubation, etc.).

Fluorescence or defluorescence of TPN/TPNH and DPN/DPNH may be employed to identify severe deficiencies of G6PD and pyruvate kinase. These reactions are the basis of simple spot tests available for screening purposes (97). Detection of milder variants and heterozygotes requires more sophisticated studies of enzyme kinetics.

REFERENCES

1. Williams, W.J., E. Beutler, A.J. Erslev and R.W. Rundles (eds.): Hematology. McGraw Hill, Inc., New York, 1972.

2. Wintrobe, M.M.: Clinical Hematology, 6th ed. Lea & Febiger, Philadelphia, 1967.

3. Harris, J.W. and R.W. Kellermeyer: The Red Cell - Production, Metabolism, Destruction: Normal and Abnormal. Harvard University Press, Cambridge, Massachusetts, 1970.

4. Van Dyke, D.: Similarity in distribution of skeletal blood flow and erythropoietic marrow. Clinical Orthopaedics 52: 37-51, 1967.

5. Weiss, L.: The Cells and Tissues of the Immune System - Structure, Functions, Interactions. Prentice-Hall, Inc., Englewood Cliffs, New Jersey, 1972.

6. Leblond, P.F., P.L. LaCelle and R.I. Weed: Cellular deformability: A possible determinant of the normal release of maturing erythrocytes from the bone marrow. Blood 37: 40-46, 1971.

7. Van Dyke, D. and N. Harris: Bone marrow reactions to trauma - Stimulation of erythropoietic marrow by mechanical disruption, fracture or endosteal curettage. Blood 34: 257-275, 1969.

8. van Bekkum, D.W., M.J. van Noord, B. Maat and K.A. Dicke: Attempts at identification of hemopoietic stem cell in mouse. Blood 38: 547-558, 1971.

9. McCulloch, E.A.: Control of hematopoiesis at the cellular level. IN Regulation of Hematopoiesis. Ed., A.S. Gordon. Appleton-Century-Crofts, 1970, p. 133-159.

10. Stohlman, F., Jr.: Aplastic anemia. Blood 40: 282-286, 1972 (editorial).

11. Labardini, J., et al.: Marrow radioiron kinetics. Haematologia (in press).

12. Bainton, D.F. and C.A. Finch: The diagnosis of iron deficiency anemia. Amer. J. Med. 37: 62-70, 1964.

13. Perutz, M.D.: The Croonian Lecture, 1968. The haemoglobin molecule. Proc. Roy. Soc. London 173: 113-140, 1969.

14. Perutz, M.F.: Stereochemistry of cooperative effects in haemoglobin. Nature 228: 726-739, 1970.

15. Stamatoyannopoulos, G., A.J. Bellingham, C. Lenfant and C.A. Finch: Abnormal hemoglobins with high and low oxygen affinity. Ann. Rev. Med. 22: 221-234, 1971

16. Jacob, H.S., A. Ruby, E.S. Overland and D. Mazia: Abnormal membrane protein of red blood cells in hereditary spherocytosis. J. Clin. Invest. 50: 1800-1805, 1971.

17. Shohet, S.B.: Hemolysis and changes in erythrocyte membrane lipids. New Eng. J. Med. 286: 577-583, 1972.

18. Race, R.R. and R. Sanger: Blood Groups in Man, 5th ed. Davis and Co., Philadelphia, 1968.

19. Pardoe, G.I.: Topochemistry of erythrocyte antigens. Nouv. Rev. Franc. Hemat. 11: 863-877, 1971.

20. Mollison, P.L.: Blood Transfusion in Clinical Medicine, 5th ed. Blackwell Scientific Publications, Oxford, Edinburgh, 1972.

21. Dern, R.J., G.J. Brewer and J.J. Wiorkowski: Studies on the preservation of human blood. II. The relationship of erythrocyte adenosine triphosphate levels and other in vitro measures to red cell storageability. J. Lab. Clin. Med. 69: 968-978, 1967.

22. Cohen, R.J., J.R. Sachs, D.J. Wicker and M.R. Conrad: Methemoglobinemia provoked by malarial chemoprophylaxis in Vietnam. New Eng. J. Med. 279: 1127-1131, 1968.

23. Finch, C.A.: Methemoglobinemia and sulfhemoglobinemia. New Eng. J. Med. 239: 470-478, 1948.

24. Jaffe, E.R.: Hereditary methemoglobinemias associated with abnormalities in the metabolism of erythrocytes. Amer. J. Med. 41: 786-798, 1966.

25. Oski, F.A. and A.J. Gottlieb: The interrelationships between red blood cell metabolites, hemoglobin, and the oxygen equilibrium curve. IN Progress in Hematology, Vol. VII. E.B. Brown and C.V. Moore (eds.). Grune and Stratton, New York, 1971, pp. 33-68.

26. Bunn, H.F.: Erythrocyte destruction and hemoglobin catabolism. Semin. Hemat. 9: 3-17, 1972.

27. Pimstone, N.R., R. Tenhunen, P.T. Seitz, H.S. Marver and R. Schmid: The enzymatic degradation of hemoglobin to bile pigments by macrophages. J. Exp. Med. 133: 1264-1281, 1971.

28. Coburn, R.F.: Endogenous carbon monoxide production. New Eng. J. Med. 282: 207-209, 1970.

29. Berlin, N.I., P.D. Berk and R.B. Howe: Disorders of bilirubin metabolism. IN Duncan's Diseases of Metabolism, 6th ed. P.K. Bondy (ed.). W.B. Saunders Co., Philadelphia, 1969, pp. 636-653.

30. Javid, J.: Human serum haptoglobins. Semin. Hemat. 4: 35-52, 1967.

31. Hershko, C., J.D. Cook and C.A. Finch: Storage iron kinetics. II. The uptake of hemoglobin iron by hepatic parenchymal cells. J. Lab. Clin. Med. 80: 624-634, 1972.

32. Muller-Eberhard, U.: Hemopexin. New Eng. J. Med. 283: 1090-1094, 1970.

33. Cook, J.D., G. Marsaglia, J.W. Eschbach, D.D. Funk and C.A. Finch: Ferrokinetics: A biologic model for plasma iron exchange in man. J. Clin. Invest. 49: 197-205, 1970.

34. Finch, C.A., K. Deubelbeiss, J.D. Cook, J.W. Eschbach, L.A. Harker, D.D. Funk, G. Marsaglia, R.S. Hillman, S. Slichter, J.W. Adamson, A. Ganzoni and E.R. Giblett: Ferrokinetics in Man. Medicine 49: 17-53, 1970.

35. Engstedt, L., S. Johansson and A. Nyberg: Estimation of human erythrocyte life-span from bilirubin turnover. J. Lab. Clin. Med. 70: 195-203, 1967.

36. Giblett, E.R., D.H. Coleman, G. Pirzio-Biroli, D.M. Donohue, A.G. Motulsky and C.A. Finch: Erythrokinetics: quantitative measurements of red cell production and destruction in normal subjects and patients with anemia. Blood 11: 291-309, 1956.

37. Viteri, F.E., J. Alvarado, D.G. Luthringer and R.P. Wood II: Hematological changes in protein calorie malnutrition. Vit. & Horm. 26: 573-615, 1968.

38. Finch, C.A.: Protein deficiency and anemia. International Society of Haematology (Proc. 12th Congress, New York City, Sept. 1968). Ed., E.R. Jaffé, New York, 1968, pp. 154-158.

39. Green, R., R. Charlton, H. Seftel, T. Bothwell, F. Mayet, B. Adams, C. Finch and M. Layrisse: Body iron excretion in man - A collaborative study. Amer. J. Med. 45: 336-353, 1968.

40. Nutritional anaemias. Report of a WHO Group of Experts. WHO Tech. Rep. Ser., No. 503, 1972.

41. Fairbanks, V.F., J.L. Fahey and E. Beutler: Clinical Disorders of Iron Metabolism, 2nd ed. Grune & Stratton, New York, 1971.

42. Pearson, H.A.: Iron-Fortified Formulas in Infancy - Commentary. The Journal of Pediatrics 79: 557-559, 1971.

43. Langer, E.E., R.G. Haining, R.F. Labbe, P. Jacobs, E.F. Crosby and C.A. Finch Finch: Erythrocyte protoporphyrin. Blood 40: 112-118, 1972.

44. Gordon, A.S.: Regulation of Hematopoiesis. Vol. I. Appleton-Century-Crofts, 1970.

45. Adamson, J.W.: The erythropoietin/hematocrit relationship in normal and polycythemic man: implications of marrow regulation. Blood 32: 597-609, 1968.

46. Card, Robert T. and M.C. Brain: The "Anemia" of Childhood - Evidence for a Physiologic Response to Hyperphosphatemia. New Eng. J. Med 288: 388-392, 1973.

47. Papayannopoulou, T. and C.A. Finch: On the in vivo action of erythropoietin: erythropoietin: A quantitative analysis. J. Clin. Invest. 51: 1179-1185, 1972.

48. Perrotta, A.L. and C.A. Finch: The polychromatophilic erythrocyte. Amer. J. Clin. Path. 57: 471-477, 1972.

49. Hillman, R.S.: Characteristics of marrow production and reticulocyte maturation in normal man in response to anemia. J. Clin. Invest. 48: 443-453, 1969.

50. Hamstra, R.D. and M.H. Block: Erythropoiesis in response to blood loss in man. J. Appl. Physiol. 27: 503-507, 1969.

51. Frenkel, E.P., M.S. McCall, J.S. Reisch and P.D. Minton: An analysis of methods for the prediction of normal erythrocyte mass. Amer. J. Clin. Path. 58: 260-273, 1972.

52. Sjöstrand, T.: Blood volume. IN Handbook of Physiology, Vol. 1. Amer. Physiol. Soc., 1962, pp. 51-62.

53. Finch, C.A. and C. Lenfant: Oxygen transport in man. New Eng. J. Med. 286: 407-415, 1972.

54. Woodson, R.D., B. Wranne and J.C. Detter: Effect of increased blood oxygen affinity on work performance of rats. J. Clin. Invest. (In press.)

55. Varat, M.A., R.J. Adolph and N.O. Fowler: Cardiovascular effects of anemia. Amer. Heart J. 83: 415-526, 1972.

56. Cook, J.D., et al.: Nutritional deficiency and anemia in Latin America: A collaborative study. Blood 38: 591-603, 1971.

57. Clarke, R., E. Topley and C.T.G. Flear: Assessment of blood-loss in civilian trauma. Lancet 1: 629-638, 1955.

58. Noble, R.P. and M.I. Gregersen: Blood volume in clinical shock. II. The extent and cause of blood volume reduction in traumatic, hemorrhagic, and burn shock. J. Clin. Invest. 25: 172-183, 1946.

59. Adamson, J. and R.S. Hillman: Blood volume and plasma protein replacement following acute blood loss in normal man. JAMA 205: 609-612, 1968.

60. Lowery, B.D., C.T. Cloutier and L.C. Carey: Electrolyte solutions in resuscitation in human hemorrhagic shock. Surg., Gynecol. Obstet. 133: 273-284, 1971.

61. Jacobs, P. and C.A. Finch: Iron for erythropoiesis. Blood 37: 220-230, 1971.

62. Finch, C.A. and J.D. Cook: Iron deficiency and its recognition. IN
    Proceedings of the IX International Congress of Nutrition (Symp. on Iron
    in Human Nutrition, Sept. 7, 1972). A. Chavez, ed. S. Karger AG, Basel,
    Switzerland (in press).

63. Hallberg, L., A. Högdahl, L. Nillson and G. Rybo: Menstrual blood loss –
    A population study. Acta Obstet. Gynec. Scandin. 45: 320-351, 1966.

64. Sölvell, L.: Oral iron therapy – side effects. IN Iron Deficiency.
    Pathogenesis, Clinical Aspects, Therapy. (Proc. Clinical Symposium on Iron
    Deficiency, Arosa, Switzerland, March, 1969). L. Hallberg, H.-G. Harweth
    and A. Vannotti, eds. Academic Press, London, 1970, pp. 573-583.

65. Sánchez-Medal, L.: The hemopoietic action of androstanes. IN Progress in
    Hematology, Vol. VII. E.B. Brown and C.V. Moore (eds.) Grune and Stratton,
    New York, 1971, pp. 111-136.

66. Safdar, S.H., S.B. Krantz and E.B. Brown: Successful immunosuppressive
    treatment of erythroid aplasia appearing after thymectomy. Brit. J.
    Haemat. 19: 435-443, 1970.

67. Adamson, J.W., J. Eschbach and C.A. Finch: The kidney and erythropoiesis.
    Amer. J. Med. 44: 725-733, 1968.

68. Huehns, E.R. and A.J. Bellingham: Disease of function and stability of
    haemoglobin. Brit. J. Haemat. 17: 1-10, 1969.

69. Eichner, E.R. and R.S. Hillman: The evolution of anemia in alcoholic
    patients. Amer. J. Med. 50: 218-232, 1971.

70. Sullivan, L.W.: Differential diagnosis and management of the patient with
    megaloblastic anemia. Amer. J. Med. 48: 609-617, 1970.

71. Herbert, V.: The five possible causes of all nutrient deficiency:
    illustrated by deficiencies of vitamin B_{12} and folic acid. Amer. J. Clin.
    Nutr. 26: 77-86, 1973.

72. Cooper, R.A. and S.J. Shattil: Mechanisms of hemolysis – the minimal red-
    cell defect. New Eng. J. Med. 285: 1514-1520, 1971.

73. Emerson, P.M.: Haemolytic anaemias: aetiology and diagnosis. Brit. J.
    Hospital Med. 6: 607-616, 1971.

74. Brain, M.D.: Microangiopathic hemolytic anemia. New Eng. J. Med. 281:
    833-835, 1969.

75. Dacie, J.V.: Autoimmune haemolytic anaemias. Brit. Med. J. 2: 381-386,
    1970.

76. Nathan, D.G. and S.B. Shohet: Erythrocyte ion transport defects and
    hemolytic anemia: "hydrocytosis" and "desiccytosis." Semin. Hematol. 7:
    381-408, 1970.

77. Edwards, E.A. and M.H. Cooley: Peripheral vascular symptoms as the initial manifestation of polycythemia vera. JAMA 214: 1463-1467, 1970.

78. Brown, S.M., H.S. Gilbert, S. Krauss and L.R. Wasserman: Spurious (relative) polycythemia: A nonexistent disease. Amer. J. Med. 50: 200-207, 1971.

79. Krantz, S.B. and L.O. Jacobson: Erythropoietin and the Regulation of Erythropoiesis. The University of Chicago Press, Chicago, 1970.

80. Thorling, E.B.: Paraneoplastic erythrocytosis and inappropriate erythropoietin production, a review. Scand. J. Haemat., Supplem. 17, 1972.

81. Adamson, J.W., G. Stamatoyannopoulos, S. Koutras, A. Lascari and J. Detter: Recessive familial erythrocytosis: Aspects of marrow regulation in two families. Blood 41: 641-652, 1973.

82. Cook, J.D.: Methods to determine plasma iron and total iron-binding capacity. IN Iron Deficiency. Pathogenesis, Clincial Aspects, Therapy (Proc. Clinical Symposium in Iron Deficiency - International Geigy Symposium, Arosa, Switzerland, March, 1969). Ed., L. Hallberg, H.-G. Harwerth and A. Vannotti, Academic Press, New York, 1970, pp. 397-407.

83. Douglas, A.S. and J.V. Dacie: The incidence and significance of iron-containing granules in human erythrocytes and their precursors. J. Clin. Path. 6: 307-313, 1953.

84. Betke, K., H.R. Marti and I. Schlicht: Estimation of small percentage of foetal hemoglobin. Nature 184: 1877-1878, 1959.

85. Huntsman, R.G., G.P. Barclay and D.M. Canning: A rapid whole blood solubility test to differentiate the sickle cell trait from sickle cell anemia. J. Clin. Path 23: 781-783, 1970.

86. Barnes, M.G., L. Komarmy and A.H. Novack: A comprehensive screening program for hemoglobinopathies. J. Amer. Med. Assoc. 219: 701-705, 1972.

87. Lau, K., C. Gottlieb, L. Wasserman and V. Herbert: Measurement of serum vitamin B-12 level using radioisotope dilution and coated charcoal. Blood 26: 202-214, 1965.

88. Hillman, R.S., M. Oakes and C.L. Finholt: Hemoglobin-coated charcoal radioassay for serum vitamin B-12. A simple modification improves intrinsic factor reliability. Blood 34: 385-390, 1969.

89. Barness, L.A., D. Young, W.J. Mellman, S.B. Kahn and W.J. Williams: Methylmalonate excretion in a patient with pernicious anemia. New Eng. J. Med. 268: 144-146, 1963.

90. Bashir, H., H. Hintenberger and B.A. Jones: Methylmalonic acid excretion in vitamin B-12 deficiency. Brit. J. Haemat. 12: 704-711, 1966.

91. Nelp, W.B., J.G. McAfee and H.M. Wagner: Single measurement of plasma radioactive B-12 as a test for pernicious anemia. J. Lab. Clin. Med. 61: 158-165, 1963.

92. Witts, L.J.: The stomach and anaemia. The Athlone Press, London, 1966.

93. Herbert, V.: Aseptic addition method for lactobacillus casei assay for folate activity in human serum. J. Clin. Path. 19: 12-16, 1966.

94. Hartman, R.C., D.E. Jenkins and A.R. Arnold: Diagnostic specificity of sucrose hemolysis test for PNH. Blood 35: 462-475, 1970.

95. Beutler, E., R.J. Dern and A.S. Alving: The hemolytic effect of Primaquine VI. An in vitro test for sensitivity of erythrocytes to primaquine. J. Lab. Clin. Med. 45: 40-50, 1955.

96. Carrell, R.W. and R. Kay: A simple method for the detection of unstable hemoglobins. Brit. J. Haem. 23: 615-619, 1972.

97. Beutler, E.: Red Cell Metabolism, A manual of biochemical methods. Grune & Stratton, New York, 1971.

GLOSSARY/INDEX